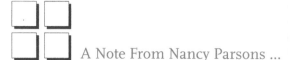
A Note From Nancy Parsons ...

D1706821

Thanks for your order of 1 copy of
Bald As A Bean. (PayPal transaction
information is enclosed.) A portion of
the proceeds from this book will go to
NAAF (National Alopecia Areata
Foundation).

I hope you enjoy "Bean".

Sincerely

Nancy

Best wishes —
Nancy Parrino

BALD AS A BEAN

By the Same Author

Morsels From The Better Mousetrap
(with Dick Amsterdam)

BALD AS A BEAN

The Experience of Sudden Hair Loss

Nancy Parsons

Bald As A Bean
The Experience of Sudden Hair Loss
Nancy Parsons

Published by Nancy L. Parsons
8 Damon Street
North Reading, MA 01864
www.nancyparsonspubs.com

ISBN: 0-9785395-0-8
Library of Congress Control Number: 2006903882

Printed in the United States of America

Photo credits:
Cover photo: Don Doyle
Back cover photo: Patty Woodbury

Parsons, Nancy L
Bald As A Bean: The Experience Of Sudden Hair Loss

To Don

Who endured the experience of sudden
hair loss—just not on his own head

CONTENTS

SPRING

INTRODUCTION

When she had run out of prescriptions and therapies and even advice to give me, Dr. Chapin gave me a compliment.

"You have an amazing attitude about this," she said. "You seem to have learned to live comfortably with a difficult situation."

Then she made a witty suggestion: "Why don't you write a book? Go on Oprah."

And with this light remark, she sailed out of the room, closing the examining room door gently behind her.

But I *was* writing—it's how a writer registers life's events, it's how a writer copes—I'd been at it since the onset of my weird adventure with hair loss. But was it a book? I thought of it simply as a process. Writing was how I made sense of a seemingly senseless and outrageous event. It was therapy of my own devising.

Bald As A Bean turns out to be the result of all that writing about all that hair business. It's a compilation of observations, annoyances, reminiscences, and the mental spelunking of a writer who happens to be losing all her hair.

Although Dr. Chapin didn't appear to know it, I wasn't as "comfortable" with that difficult situation as she seemed to think. The brave face I assumed in her office was often just a mask—and a comedic Greek mask at that, the alter ego of the mask of tragedy. In the beginning, I used this mask to hide my true feelings of horror, embarrassment, and panic; at some point though, the mask dropped away and I did find acceptance and the sense of peace that comes with it.

There are several messages here—several points that I want to make: that hair is an emotional issue in the best of times and that the loss of hair can be traumatic. And I want to make it plain that even in the grip of trauma, there are choices. While hair loss is certainly an emotional issue for women, it is for men as well. The person experiencing sudden hair loss, whether through chemotherapy or alopecia or some idiopathic cause, may have no control over the baldness, but each does have choices about dealing with the problems. I came to understand that my choices not only affected my outlook, but they also influenced how others handled my baldness. In time I came to see that my experience had something in common with the grieving process that was identified and deconstructed several decades ago—a process that runs through denial and anger to ultimate acceptance. In the end, I think I made the choice to accept being bald. The choice makes the difference between illness and health.

AUTUMN

BALD AS A BEAN

A VERY BAD HAIR DAY

There is one true thing that could be said about my hair: it was thick. It could also be said that it was fine and straight, that it had no body, that it refused to hold curl and that it was the color of the mouse you find dead in the trap in the morning. But at least it was thick. Then came alopecia.

Of course I didn't know it was alopecia; I just thought ... "Omigod!"

One morning in the shower my hand came away from my shampoo-covered head dragging a hank of sudsy hair, and my heart nearly dropped through the drain. I stood under the showerhead with a fistful of my own hair and a heart that was banging like old radiator pipes.

Well, I've always lost some hair in the shower, I told myself shakily. I seem to shed it like a dog in summertime. Hair on the bathroom floor, hair in my brush—no matter— it still sprouted on my head in a mat so deep that it required a full ten to fifteen minutes with a dryer. Thick and layered as a Labrador Retriever's coat, my hair held dampness for hours. Now here I was, losing it in wads. I was terrified.

This simply isn't happening, I said. I'm a big believer in denial.

The next morning, though, I emerged wet-headed from the shower to discover that the hair on the back of my head had knotted itself into hideous rats' nests. Two of these snarls came away easily in the comb, leaving glossy patches on my scalp where they had once been rooted.

Denial was no longer an option. Action was called for.

I reasoned that a dermatologist would be the best doctor to call—after all, isn't hair just a variant of skin?— so I put in a call to Dr. Chapin who had treated me off and on for rashes and moles, and I ran smack into her receptionist. (Is there an employment agency for medical receptionists? I want to know this. Do they have to pass a course in abruptness training before they can be hired into a medical office?) I forced my voice to be light, aiming for a casual "it's-always-something-isn't it?" tone, which came off as sort of a nervous whinny.

"I seem to be losing my hair. Does Dr. Chapin treat that sort of problem?"

"Oh yes," the receptionist assured me. And then she named an appointment date that was six weeks away.

"You could be bald by then," taunted the voice that talks to me inside my head.

"Can't you give me anything sooner?" The casual tone evaporated. I heard my own voice escalate into a range that only dogs hear. I've never been terribly assertive but now I gasped, "Isn't there a cancellation or something?"

We haggled and finally settled on a time that was still much farther off than I wished (what I wanted was an appointment in about twenty minutes) but this criminally distant date was the best I could negotiate. And it would have to do.

My hair continued to deciduate. As I drove my car, long strands fell onto my shoulders; these I'd deposit on the passenger seat until I reached the next stop light, when I'd roll down the window and dispose of them. Every sweater and jacket displayed a shawl of hair. In case you don't know, polar fleece is mad for hair; each strand embeds in the fibers and has to be extracted one at a time. I began to feel like a hirsute Typhoid Mary every time I walked into the kitchen.

One morning, after another disastrous combing session, I called Dr. Chapin's office and begged the receptionist for an appointment. She relented. I had an appointment for four days later. My relief was vast.

By the time I'd waited the four days, combed out at least two more pounds of hair, driven to the office, waited for forty minutes, read back copies of *Architectural Digest* and *InStyle*, and finally been ushered into the examining room, I was shaking. I could barely hold the pen to fill out a questionnaire on my hair history. As I looked at my own spidery writing quavering above and below the lines that had been provided for my answers, I realized how troubled I really was.

WELCOME TO ALOPECIA

Dr. Chapin has obviously seen a lot of hysterical people who think they are losing their hair.

"Is your hair just breaking or is it coming out at the roots?"

"The roots."

'Hmmmm."

I bend my head penitently while she fluffs through my hair. This cursory examination is followed with another thoughtful "Hmmmmm."

Sudden hair loss, she explains, is often the result of a trauma that may have happened some months earlier—usually about five months earlier. Stress, she says, is very often the cause. Then she tells me a story of the hair loss cases she'd seen when she was a resident in California and had treated a number of Cambodian boat people. These refugees, she recalls, had survived the terrors of the Khymer Rouge, of jungle mazes, of perilous passages in unseaworthy boats—not to mention malnutrition and disease—and had finally reached America and freedom, only to have their hair fall out once they had reached safety. There you are! Stress! Stress is the moral of her story and she plays it like a triumphant ace.

She is keen to know if there has been any stress in my life.

I assure her my life is and has been stress-free, but I remind her of the case of Lyme disease that I'd had the preceding summer—a case that she herself had diagnosed and treated.

"Hmmmmm."

"Well, it *could* be from Lyme," she says carefully, "although that is highly unlikely. Are you sure you're not stressed?" She smiles encouragingly as if to let me know it is safe to confide my secrets to her.

I shake my head firmly. There have been times in my life when stress was a constant pressure; I am all too familiar with the clutch of anxiety that congeals in the chest and makes it hard to breathe. If there is one thing I understand it is stress. I also know when it is absent.

She continues to smile but a couple of shades of doubt slightly darken her expression. Well, *this* is denial; I can almost hear her thinking, and a big case, too.

She returns to her perusal of my scalp. I hear her murmur alopecia areata, which I misunderstand as irriatata. Some sort of scalp irritation, I think. Good. Irritations can be grotty, but they can be cleared up with a few treatments of an antibiotic. Write out a prescription and we'll be all set.

"Well, in any case," says Dr. Chapin, rising from her inspection, "we have to run a few tests before we can reach any solid conclusion about this."

As an interim treatment though, she prescribes cortisone shampoo and cortisone drops. These I embrace like a drowning woman grabs for a rope. Twice daily I faithfully launder my weak hair and drip the medicine onto my scalp, but the harvest of falling hair continues unabated.

It takes several weeks and a battery of blood tests before Dr. Chapin makes a firm diagnosis. When the tests come back negative for such problems as a misfiring thyroid or out-of-whack hormones, her original suspicions are confirmed—alopecia areata. The enemy is named.

As I wait for the word from the lab, I think of little else than my hair. It's understandable since there is always at least one newly-released strand brushing my cheek or swaying tauntingly in front of my eyes.

But once the condition is declared, I start to learn incredible things about myself—about my physical self and my emotional self. My physical self feels fine. There is no loss of energy, no lethargy, no aches or pains. My emotional self isn't as robust. In fact, it is pretty shaky.

"Alopecia," claims the National Alopecia Foundation, "is not life threatening, but it is life changing."

The assertion proves both prophetic and true.

DECIDUATING

The days march into deep November. The sugar maple on the front lawn and the Norway maple in the backyard are shedding leaves in earnest. The yard is a thick mat of yellow. Indoors, I am deciduating, too.

Dr. Chapin explains, as she riffles through my head, scattering hairs all over the office floor, that the hair that is going to come out *will* come out. Tender treatment won't preserve what has been deprived of nutrients. Nevertheless, she bans the use of hairbrushes, hair dryers, hot rollers, curling irons—all favorite tools of mine—as well as barrettes, clips, clamps and elastic bands. The single hair implement I am allowed is a wide-toothed comb. This I am instructed to use very gingerly.

Every morning before my shower—and to relieve our overtaxed shower drain—I run my fingers through my hair, ruffling and fluffing and pulling lightly. Hair rains to the floor while outside, the late autumn winds blow through the yellow leaves on our trees, carrying the loose ones to the ground. In the autumn sadness of dark, damp days, I alternately rake leaves and wipe up my own fallen hair.

But despite the kid-glove treatment, the shower's pounding water releases what seems like pounds of hair. I bend over constantly to swoop great seaweed swales of it out of the strainer over the drain. And when I comb out my damp hair, the prescribed wide tooth comb harvests a horrifying crop.

I ask Dr. Chapin if I will lose all my hair before new growth starts. "Not necessarily," she says rather evasively. Then she adds a cryptic postscript: "You may not lose it *all*."

The most pressing questions I have for Dr. Chapin is: Will new hair grow? And how soon?

Her answers are maddeningly vague. She refuses, almost perversely it seems to me, to give me any good news. Or even much glimmer of hope.

"Sometimes with alopecia areata, hair *does* grow back." She has a habit of smiling while she speaks, and she is smiling away sweetly as she says this, but her tone has a hedging quality.

"One rule of thumb," she says, "is the younger you are when you lose your hair, the less chance you have of regrowth."

This is great news!

"Whew! Then I am all set," I joke weakly. At age sixty-two, I certainly can't be considered young. I fire off next question:

"When can I expect some regrowth?"

But Dr. Chapin won't say. A Mona Lisa smile, a shrug and no commitment. But she does offer another sliver of enlightenment. "When the hair follicles decide to wake up and the hair grows back, it is often different than the hair it replaces. It may be curly instead of straight. Or it may be quite dark instead of light. But sometimes this hair will change again."

I decide I don't care what my new hair looks like: it will be welcome in whatever color or texture.

But for now my focus is on the incumbent hair. And I want the deciduation to stop. Every morning I wake, hoping this will be the day. Please, let this be the day that no hair falls on the bathroom floor when I shake out the loose stuff. Please, no more sopping strands sweeping along toward the shower drain. Please, just let it stop and I will go to the hairdresser and get some stylish short cut that will hide the balding spots and this will tide me over until the new crop grows in.

Eventually the maples stand bare on the lawn, their leaves raked and composted. My hair continues to fall. Resigned, I keep sweeping.

DON

This is what he has always said: "Will you still love me if I go bald?"

Don frets constantly about this thinning hair, but I could never figure out why. Nor could I understand why my assurances that I will continue to adore him never seem to appease his uncertainty. Now I'm the one with thinning hair—with more than thinning hair, with actual bald spots—and I can't get outside myself long enough to consider how my husband is handling it.

"I think I'm losing my hair," I confide to him one day.

"Oh thank God!" he gasps. Then, answering my goggling stare, he adds, I thought I was just imagining it."

"Imagining what?"

"That you were going bald. I went to kiss the back of your head one day and I actually kissed a glossy spot. I was horrified. I thought you were exercising too much and were losing your hair because of it."

"You didn't say anything."

"You didn't say you were losing your hair."

I hadn't known that I was balding on the top and back of my head, since I don't usually see those locations. How long had he been viewing these bald spots? But one morning I discover I have lost considerable amounts of hair on my temples. My heart accelerates. I can see actual bare scalp above my ears. I'd seen my wet hair plastered flat to my head, but I'd never actually seen the skull. I've had hair on my head as far back as I could remember, and I certainly had no idea that there were glossy spots on public view.

But I still didn't give much thought to my husband's reaction to this development until our young financial advisor raises the question during a portfolio review.

"How is Don taking this?" Mike wants to know, after he has extended his unqualified sympathy about my diagnosis. ("Well, thank God!" he said, "I thought it was something much worse.")

Suddenly I realize I haven't been totally in touch with how Don is taking it. It had seemed like my issue—a totally self-absorbing matter—but it becomes clear in a flash that a man whose wife is going bald is certainly going to have issues of his own.

I pause to search for an answer to give Mike. Then I say the only true thing I can think of: "Every morning when I wake up he says to me, 'Good morning, Beautiful.' I know that I am about as beautiful as a boiled egg, but I really appreciate having him say it."

"I am sure," Michael replies generously, and I think genuinely, "that to him you are very beautiful."

And then my throat closes, and I can't speak reliably for a few seconds.

HUMBERTO

The gods had been shooting craps with hair for my entire life and then, to add insult to injury, I fall in with someone named Humberto. It begins when Dr. Chapin opens the examining room door and prepares to leave. Then she seems to have a second thought and looks back in at me.

"You could always get a wig, you know. It might help over the holidays." Then—whisk—she is gone.

Her nurse bustles back in with two prescriptions and Humberto's pamphlet, *Thinning hair, problem hair, hair replacement.* I make an appointment over the phone with Humberto's receptionist, who clearly hasn't passed the seventh grade. I hear her shift her chewing gum to the other side of her mouth before saying: "Thursday eve-a-ning. Seven a-'clock, that's when he sees people for ... special ... a-poyments. An' by-the-way, ya betta gimme ya numbah."

Humberto's hair salon not only smells like every other hair salon in the world, but it also has the same messy clutter of cans, hairbrushes, and back copies of *Vogue*, *Redbook*, and *People*. Somehow I thought this place would be different. I thought it would have an antiseptic, doctor's office sort of feel. But on this Thursday eve-a-ning, I humbly sit and wait my turn with the great man Humberto. From a shelf that runs around all four walls of the shop, Styrofoam mannequins wearing frazzled wigs and identical, insipid expressions simper down at me. I reach for a dog-eared copy of *People* and hide from their gazes.

"Hmmm, yes." Humberto's professional fingers fluff through my hair. "Are you on ... " he pauses delicately, "chemotherapy?"

I explain.

Humberto waltzes into another room and returns with a wig—which he carefully calls a unit. Delicacy apparently forbids Humberto to use the word wig. The, er, unit looks very much like my own hair. More accurately, it looks a lot like my hair used to look—a thick, light ash brown pageboy. Its familiarity is somehow comforting.

"First," proclaims Humberto, "we put on a cap. This is to keep the unit clean."

He rips open a cellophane package and shakes out a skullcap. Then he gathers my hair, pulling it back, and tugs the flesh-colored nylon cap down to my ears in preparation for the unit.

Humberto ventures a joke. "We look like we're going to rob a bank, yes?"

From Humberto's mirror, Tommy Hedberg looks back at me. Memory hits instant rewind and it is 1949.

My elementary school is in the throes of a ringworm epidemic. Once a week each classroom of children is marched down to the school nurse's office where one by one we enter her dark supply closet to have our scalps searched under a black light. It is terrifying. The nurse's very appearance at the door to the classroom, extending her beckoning finger, starts my heart racing, and by the time I approach this dark door, I am breathing in short, rapid bursts of near-hysteria.

The nurse's savage fingers frantically plunder our scalps, pulling our hair into rats and tangles until she is satisfied we are vermin-free. Then she dismisses us from the closet. Reeling from the sudden light and weak-kneed with relief, I stagger back into the glare of her office while the next hapless child brushes past and is absorbed by the ominous dark.

Every week three or four boys in the school fail the inspection. They disappear for a few days, presumably to be purged and shriven with horrible medications. When they return, it is with shaved heads under skullcaps made from their mothers' nylon stockings. No girl ever gets ringworm, but I have dreaded images of being the first. The shame and mortification of it is almost more than I can contemplate.

The ringworm scourge comes closest to our third grade class when Tommy Hedberg vanishes. Tommy is a plump, mild boy whose fat cheeks shine red. He is absent for a week. When he returns, it is—oddly—in the middle of the day.

Returning from lunch, we find him sitting at his desk by the windows, staring fixedly outside. Except he isn't really seeing anything. His eyes are full of tears and his cheeks are redder and shinier than ever. His mother, Mrs. Hedberg, who is clearly the author of Tommy's shiny plumpness, stands beside his desk giving him gentle reassurance and encouragement. I like her housedress and her sensible oxfords and the fact that she has accompanied Tommy and stays with him as long as she can. And I keenly feel Tommy's humiliation, but I am seven or eight-years-old. I haven't yet gained the maturity and grace to know the right thing to say so I avert my eyes and offer no word of comfort or support. It seems safest to simply pretend that neither Tommy nor his poor head is there. It is a reaction I will eventually come to experience myself, only I will not be the one doing the pretending.

Now, staring at my reflection in Humberto's mirror, I think, "I am Tommy Hedberg."

In two more seconds, though, I am looking out from under the bangs of an elaborate pageboy, Tommy Hedberg has vanished, and so does the woman I've become in the past weeks. The frail halo of deciduating hair is hidden and instant self-possession is bestowed. Humberto, I can see, was pleased with himself. And for my part, there is some relief.

"Yes," I agree, "I think this is the one."

I wear the wig, excuse me—the unit—home and model it for a bemused Donald. He doesn't seem to know what to say. My head is beginning to ache, perhaps from the pinching skullcap.

In the bathroom mirror, I stare at the unit and at my face under it. How had I ever thought it looked like my own hair? I look like I'm going to a costume party tricked out as Barbra Streisand.

"Come on, Babs," I tell the wig. "It's going to take a lot more nerve than I have right now to waltz with you in public."

A large carton has arrived from L.L. Bean with a bounty of things ordered for Christmas. Into this now empty carton I pack the wig carefully, tucking tissue paper around the base of the smirking Styrofoam mannequin that Humberto threw in "for free" while I was writing the check for $365. The Tommy Hedberg ringworm cap gets tossed in just before I weave the flaps of the box closed over Babs's part. At the back of the closet where my long gowns and Don's tuxedo hang, I park the carton with my new hair; then I crawl out of the closet backwards and go to find the aspirin bottle.

HOPE AND EXPECTATION

In the autumn days I begin to develop a theory. It pushes up into my mind with the force of a sprouting tulip bulb. I begin to think of it as "The Seasons Theory." It goes something like this:

I will lose my hair as the trees lose their leaves in autumn. There will be a dormant period (winter) and then spring will come and—*voila!*—new growth! The trees will put out new leaves. Flowers and grass will push up through the scumbled brown earth. And on my head, hair will begin to grow. It will just be little sprouts at first, of course, but in the heat and energy of summer, it will grow with real vigor. I see myself mixing Miracle Gro for my potted impatiens plants and although I won't, of course, be putting Miracle Gro on my head (ha ha), the warm season that encourages tomato crops and sends zucchini vines rampaging over the other garden inhabitants will also be encouraging my new hair.

I will have a year of inconvenient hair issues, I figure. And this will be all right. I can handle this temporary condition somehow, but when autumn rolls around again, with Christmas right behind it, I will have a fine new crop of locks just in time for the holiday parties. Perhaps it will be curly. Wouldn't that be fun! Or perhaps it will be white and thick and I will cut it in a pixie cap.

Okay. A year is a long time, but it isn't forever. If I have to, I can wait.

GOOGLING

Alopecia areata. The subject has the same fascination for me as a terrible auto accident might. Some dark part of my psyche wants to examine it, to take in every gristly detail, but at the same time, it is so horrifying and repellent that I'm afraid to look. So for several weeks after the diagnosis, I resist Googling. While part of me wants to surf the Internet to research every detail of my new disease, I am also afraid of what I'll find. Like looking at the auto accident, I am both attracted and repelled.

Like many people, I am not immune to suggestion, and this knowledge also keeps me from Googling. I'm really afraid that if I begin to learn more about this alopecia thing, I will develop symptoms that I don't actually have or that I probably wouldn't develop if I didn't know about them. For a graphic example of how this behavior works, I need to look no further than my husband, Don.

Don looked up from his drawing board one day—coming back to reality after a long immersion in an illustration project—to find a talk show in progress on the

TV. Don became instantly intrigued because he recognized many of the symptoms the show's participants were discussing in himself. Ridged fingernails, irritability, an overwhelming desire to sleep. Don watched avidly. At last the cause of these symptoms was revealed: candida albicans. For two days Don walked around under the pall of this distressing diagnosis until he finally decided he must learn more. After a trip to the Boston Public Library, he learned that candida albicans is a vaginal yeast infection, and therefore a malady for which he was singularly unsuited. His symptoms cleared right up.

Eventually, Pandora-like curiosity defeats my fear. I settle down to a Googling session, determined to learn more about this curious thing called alopecia areata.

Item A.

One of the first Web sites to come up is the National Alopecia Areata Foundation—www.NAAF.org. Here I get a concise explanation of my new disease. I learn it is "a highly unpredictable, autoimmune skin disease" that affects approximately 1.7% of the population. Alopecia totalis means a total loss of the hair on the scalp. Alopecia universalis is a complete loss of body hair. Since I have lost considerable body hair—arms and underarms, legs and even toe beards, those silly tufts of hair that sprout out of great toes, I conclude I have alopecia areata universalis. If I eventually lose all my hair, I will qualify for the Alopecia Ultimate: alopecia areata totalis universalis.

Well, I never liked doing things halfway.

NAAF has a helpful list of frequently asked questions and offers one of the most succinct and true statements I have ever read about the disease: "Although not life-threatening, alopecia areata is most certainly life-altering."

Item B. — People with alopecia are called Alopecians.

Odd. I figured they'd be called Alopeciacs.

Item C. — Princess Caroline of Monaco, Al Pacino, and Faye Dunaway are famous Alopecians. I add my own gloomy postscript to the list: E.T., Sigourney Weaver's character in *Alien II*, and Gollum in *Lord of the Rings*.

Item D. — Alopecia is a fourteenth-century Latin word derived from alopekia, which refers to the patchy, hairless areas sometimes seen on a fox.

Item E. — Someone has developed an alopecian Ken doll, a bald companion for Barbie, who presumably still sports a thick mane.

Item F. — The name for fine body hair is vellus hair.

Google sends me reeling off to amazing sites that cater to the bald and about-to-be-bald. A Google link, for which I will forever be grateful, landed me on the site for Headcovers.com.

This site offers sixteen pages of women's hats, turbans, and scarves. Each is featured with descriptive copy and with a photo that can be enlarged. Color swatches are generous and true. The company also has specific offerings for children and men. And they have an amazing array of wigs, all very reasonably priced.

Through most of the autumn I am able to wear civilian baseball caps, allowing fringes and spit curls of hair to poke beneath the brims. But in time the gaps at the backs of the caps become peepholes to my baldness. Traditional baseball hats began to feel precarious. Without my customary thick mat of hair to fill out the caps, they begin to feel slippery and insubstantial. I find the Headcovers site just about the time all my hats are beginning to feel like badly fitting dentures. The caps they offer and that I ordered fit snugly and comfortably. The company states that all their hats are guaranteed to provide full head coverage—a feature I come to appreciate and rely on. And they are reasonably stylish.

"I like your hat," says a woman I encounter in a store. "Where did you get it? L.L. Bean?"

"I got it online."

She is persistent. "Where exactly? It looks like that cap Tom Brady was wearing after the Super Bowl."

I sigh. "Look," I say. "All my hair has fallen out. I got this special hat on a Web site that caters to bald women."

I have to hand it to her. She never misses a beat. "Well, it looks fantastic! So smart!" And away she sweeps.

The Headcovers folks truly understand the special emotional and physical needs of the customer experiencing sudden hair loss, and they make it possible to get product within twenty-four hours (many customers are delighted and relieved to pay for the special services).

While I'm still in the heart-in-the-throat stage, I order two soft turbans and a newsboy style cap. Eventually I will send for a lace trimmed sleep cap, a second newsboy's cap, two baseball caps, and a turban that looks like a tied scarf. I also order a wig, which I look upon as temporary hair—but that is a subject and a story all its own.

THANKSGIVING

Our Thanksgiving celebration is at my sister's lake house.

"We're having two turkeys," Meg proclaims. "I am cooking one inside on the woodstove and Dave is deep frying the other one outside. We'll have a turkey competition and everyone can vote on the best-tasting turkey."

It was a good Thanksgiving—cold, but bright and clear. The men gather outside around Dave's deep fat fryer, talking sports, talking politics, who knows, but definitely talking turkey. Inside the lake house kitchen Meg bastes and chops while Abby, Joyce, and I catch up on current events; my thinning hair is among the topics.

Both turkeys are delicious, but the competition ends in a dead heat.

"For dark meat," proclaimed my son Jamie diplomatically, "the fried turkey is best, but the cookstove turkey has the best white meat."

Thus both turkey cooks win.

With Thanksgiving, the starting gun of the holiday season is fired.

And now begins an especially awkward time for me. It's the one season of the year when my party clothes get a workout; but when you are going bald, a party dress and strappy shoes just aren't sufficiently redemptive. As I bring out the Christmas decorations and set electric candles in all the windows, I begin to grow increasingly nervous.

A BIT PLAYER

Impending baldness regenerates some feelings I haven't had since early adolescence, when I believed that every other person was looking at me critically. Short of wearing a sandwich board with, I AM LOSING MY HAIR, emblazoned in 96-point Helvetica Black, I couldn't feel more conspicuous or uncomfortable.

Even so, I decide I won't stay sealed away by my own fireside. I am determined to go about my natural routine, but I realize this will require some serious coping strategies.

So I begin by trying to tell people about my difficulty before they have the chance to observe it for themselves— and draw their own, uninformed conclusions. The holidays, as always, bring a higher-than-usual number of social invitations, and I discover I am more comfortable if folks know about my problem before a gathering so they don't have to speculate. So I make a few delicate calls ahead to hosts and certain guests ...

"I just wanted to warn you ... "

"I'm fine really, but I didn't want you to be shocked when you see me ... "

"Just thought I'd tell you that if I'm wearing a wig Saturday night, it's still me under it."

Of course, each excuse opens me up to the sort of confessional stuff I hate. And then I have to listen to the expressions of horror and sympathy extended by the person I've called. There are condolences to be endured and accepted. There are thanks to be given by me for the concern expressed. There are assurances, again given by me, that I will be fine, just fine thank you—really! Finally there are the endless questions about why.

Not everyone requires an explanation, I figure. And it just isn't practical anyway. I certainly can't phone every potential guest in advance of an open house, for instance, to prepare them for how I'm going to look. Nor can I sweep through someone's front door and make a general announcement to a houseful of slight acquaintances that I am losing my hair, damn it; but here I am anyway, and I'm just delighted to see everyone. I've taken to wear a faux fur Santa Claus hat to functions, aiming for light-hearted, festive touch. But it's hard keeping the thing on during the whole event even though I'm sweating prodigiously into the pouff of white fake fur around the brim.

Then there's the issue of total strangers. This is difficult, too. I'm finding my baseball cap isn't quite covering the bald spot that is growing on the back of my head. There's that sort of peephole just above the adjustable strap, which gives people standing behind me in supermarket lines a clear view of my baldness. And what else do they have to do anyway, but stare at my condition and speculate idly, "What's wrong with her?"

This is bothering me. I have to talk to myself sharply about this. It's really a place where I need some therapy.

And so I'm developing a mantra—a quotation I remember from somewhere—"I am just a bit player in somebody else's movie."

I don't know why, but it seems to help.

BALD AS A BEAN

WINTER

BALD AS A BEAN

EMERGENCY

Character is not made in a crisis; it is only exhibited.
Anonymous

Alopecia areata is now an emergency for me, in the spiritual sense. When I break down the word emergency into its components, I find "emerge and see. The usual meaning takes a sharp right turn. The dangerous aspects of an emergency soften and there's a promise of growth and spiritual awakening. A spiritual emergency signals that something new is about to pop through into consciousness. I figure if I stay alert—if I pay attention—then I might be privileged to witness this birth. So I'm trying to see that this spiritual emergency can be a time of personal transformation.

Alopecia areata isn't a crisis in the way a severed femoral artery is an emergency. It isn't the diagnosis of cancer or news of a blocked artery ... still, I am scared and shaken. What will happen? What is going to emerge?

IRRITATION THERAPY

On the first weekday after New Year's I am in Dr. Chapin's office early, eager for her examination and avid for the next step she'll take in our mutual struggle with my drifting hair. I've lost considerably more hair over the holidays, but just how much is made dramatically clear when I hear Dr. Chapin's involuntary gasp. She recovers quickly though, and moves right in to paw through my sick locks and examine my scalp.

"Hmmmm, yes. Alopecia areata, definitely."

Dr. Chapin straightens up and continues briskly, "Well, we're going to try a few more things."

She outlines a routine that will require me to anoint my head with a variety of unguents and gunks, being careful to wash some of them off before I apply others and admonishing me to keep others on for prescribed amounts of time. I am slightly bewildered but determined to follow her directions.

There is something called tar that I am to wear all night. This stops me, and my mind drifts to consider head tar while Dr. Chapin goes on talking. I envision a thick, black substance like road tar that I daub on with a stick. I also envision myself heading into the bedroom wearing this emulsion and smelling like a new road on a summer day. I see myself approaching the unsuspecting Donald, who is propped up in bed reading. He is a mild man, Don is, and quick to leap to the most dramatic and deadly conclusions in any new situation. Heavens knows what will happen when a tar-headed bedmate shows up and slips in next to him.

But I manage to kick this image aside, and I swallow bravely and promise. "Anything you say. I'll do whatever it takes."

Dr. Chapin explains that some of the medications will irritate my scalp.

"There is a theory that irritation stimulates hair growth," she says. "In France they have actually had some success regrowing hair by applying poison ivy to the scalp." She smiles. "The FDA hasn't approved that here."

I try to picture it. I am morbidly sensitive to poison ivy, and I try to balance the trade-offs between new hair and the hideous hurting itch of a vicious two-week case of poison ivy. But Dr. Chapin is talking again and writing busily.

In moments I am clutching prescriptions for the pharmacist and a page of directions for me. I reel out of her office, and head for the drugstore, pressing a little harder than necessary on the accelerator out of eagerness to begin my medication routine—a program that will surely be my salvation. In my pocket is a new appointment card that instructs me to return to Dr. Chapin's office in one month.

Anthralin cream, tretinoin cream—also known as Retin A—and Rogaine for Women are now part of my daily routine of cortisone drops and shampoo.

The pharmacist raises his eyebrows as he reads the script for Retin A.

"You'll need permission from your insurance carrier for this," he says. "We'll have to get your doctor to contact them."

The HMO doesn't approve of Retin A, a substance used primarily to treat acne. Acne, they probably think, is something a patient will outgrow, given time, and the HMO isn't about to help out with something as frivolous and cosmetic as acne. Arguments from Dr. Chapin's office can't budge them on this score, and so a tube of tretinoin cream is going to cost me one hundred dollars.

The anthralin adds another thirty-five dollars to the bill, and a month's supply of Rogaine for Women—now available over the counter—costs forty.

Alopecia areata doesn't come cheap.

I develop an immediate aversion to Rogaine for Women. I'm reading the instructions and disclaimers on the package, and it looks to me like the success rate for Rogaine is pretty slim. Of the manufacturer's six reasons not to use the product, I possess five.

Rogaine for Women is to be applied twice daily at intervals of at least four hours. An application is not to be followed by any washing of hair or scalp. The treatments are dispensed through a rubber nippled cap; I am to daub this nipple on the bare spots—in my case, most of my head—and stand back, waiting to enjoy new hair.

The dreaded tar, which turns out to be the Retin A, is actually not unpleasant. It's a cooling, ivory cream—not black and gooey—and is fairly odorless. I feel better about wearing this emulsion to bed. I rub it into my scalp and tie a cotton bandana over my head, wondering how badly the stuff will stain.

Each morning I wash the tar out of my head with cortisone shampoo. Then I slip out of the shower still wearing the shampoo and sit for fifteen minutes while the cortisone works its charms. Back into the shower to rinse, then out of the shower to dry my hair and apply anthralin; fifteen more minutes to wait for the anthralin to percolate. Then into the shower once more to wash it off. This makes a total of three trips through the shower in fairly close order, with time in between to let the medication of the moment do its work. When my hair is dry—what remains of it anyhow—I have a go with cortisone drops, and when *that* dries, I break out the Rogaine for Women.

In this way I pass one of the coldest and darkest months of the winter.

My head grows red and burned looking. My scalp looks as if it had been seared on a barbeque. Then brown scabs form like a dark cradle cap. I'm grateful for scarves and caps which hide my diseased-looking pate. If irritation jumpstarts hair growth, I should be brushing my new locks very soon now. But peering dubiously at the sad head reflected in the mirror indicates no reason for optimism. My own head reminds me of the blueberry fields of Maine. Barrens, they are called, and with good reason, for they are brown and red, stubbled, and sere. Still, these burned fields produce a bounty of berries.

So I sigh and tell myself, "This is what healing looks like."

WHY?

Eight out of ten people who hear about my condition want to know why it's happening. Then they demand to know what can be done about it. Finally, they want to know *if* and when my hair will grow back.

Their reactions to my explanations—"no one knows and no, nothing, and I don't know when or even if it will grow back"—are met with fishy, suspicious stares. The unspoken message I'm getting is that clearly I haven't tried hard enough. I just haven't seen the right specialists; we live, after all, within minutes of Boston, seat of some of the finest medical centers in the world. Very few people I share my problem with would be prepared to accept it as calmly as I am apparently doing. We live in the Fix-It Age— the Age of Something Must Be Done. Few I share with would take this situation lying down.

The cause or causes of alopecia areata are unclear, and it has no known cure. Furthermore, there aren't any approved drugs that reverse the condition. This is a state-of-affairs that many people have trouble accepting.

"The hair follicles have gone to sleep," I try to explain, using the lay term borrowed from Dr. Chapin. "Something happens—some trigger—and the blood supply to the follicles shuts down."

What in fact happens is that the immune system cells called white blood cells attack the rapidly growing cells in the hair follicles that are in charge of hair production. The hair follicles then shrink in size and slow down their hair manufacturing tasks. The news isn't all bad, though; for some reason, the stem cells that continually supply the follicle with new cells seems to be impervious to the shutting down process, leaving open the potential and promise for hair to regrow.

The explanation why white blood cells suddenly attack is fuzzy. It seems to be a combination of things, including a genetic predisposition to some sort of trigger, which could be a virus or something in the individual's environment.

So what is the "thing" that happened to me? What was the trigger?

I don't know. I tend to blame a case of Lyme disease I had the summer before alopecia areata set in. If Lyme is certifiably responsible for some cases of rheumatoid arthritis, it seems reasonable to me that it can also trigger alopecia areata. To further bolster this theory, I need only recall Dr. Chapin's explanation that hair starts falling out from five to seven months *after* a trigger. My bout with Lyme disease occurred in June and my hair loss began in November.

But even this Lyme disease explanation fails to completely satisfy the pitying individual and I find myself still facing the fishy stare.

It is important to realize that alopecia areata comes in a variety of styles—or more accurately, degrees of severity. Many people have one or several small or large balding patches on their skulls, and this too is alopecia. In its most dramatic form, alopecia areata causes total hair loss over the entire body.

Alopecia areata, indeed all autoimmune diseases as far as I can tell, are medical mysteries. But like my friends who believe in magic bullets, I would like to have one. And I'm hoping Dr. Chapin will have some trick that reverses this hair loss and maybe even one more bullet that will bring on fresh growth.

NO MAGIC BULLETS

The best thing that can be said for present treatments of alopecia areata is that some can grow hair—temporarily. Temporary isn't good enough for most folks. It certainly isn't for me. Moreover, there is the knowledge that the disease is still there, an invisible phantom—just below the surface of the skin—and no magic bullet has been found to wipe out the phantom. Nevertheless, we can come at alopecia areata with some weapons; after all, David slew Goliath with a slingshot. Who knows? Maybe one or more of these pebbles will help.

Corticosteroids are sometimes used to treat various autoimmune diseases. These are powerful anti-inflammatory drugs, formulated to mimic the hormone cortisol, which the body produces naturally. Corticosteroids, when given orally, suppress the immune system. Why this should work, I have no idea.

Corticosteriods, available in several forms, are a major source of treatment. Local injections of cortisone directly into bald patches will produce hair in about four weeks. Sometimes a single injection can excite the growth of a full head of hair, but it is more common for half-dollar-sized patches to sprout at the injection sites. Whether or not the new hair will stick around is anybody's guess. It is as likely to wither at the root and atrophy as to turn into brushable locks.

Ointments, shampoos, and liquids that are applied topically offer other ways to administer cortisone. Because they aren't as strong as injections, however, they are less likely to germinate hair. Some topical ointments containing steroids are rubbed directly on the afflicted areas. These seem to operate best in combination with other therapies such as minoxidil and anthralin.

Minoxidil is best known by its popular name Rogaine. It works best when the hair follicles are small, localized and are just failing to produce to their full potential.

Anthralin, also known as Psoriatec or tar, is most often used to treat psoriasis. It is considered short-treatment therapy, since long exposures bring about skin irritation.

Prednisone taken orally is also a treatment option for alopecia areata. It is not a treatment of frequent choice because of its dramatic side effects, and in the end, like the other treatments, the hair growth it generates will be lost when the medicine is stopped.

THE MANGE STAGE

I seem to have selective hair loss but I don't know what is driving the selection process. Both temples are now bald and glossy. If the back of my head were a clock's face, I would have round bare patches at eleven and two. I look like a dog with mange but am reminded that the origin of the word alopecia refers to the patchy places sometimes seen on fox.

For a while a little baseball cap covered the bald spots because I am retaining the hair around the edges of my skull, like a tonsured monk. But now the hair loss is creeping lower and the space at the back of the ball cap reveals a bald skull. I am told that hair loss from chemotherapy can happen all at once. My hair loss from alopecia is happening more gradually and it's happening patchily.

I have designer baldness.

DANCING WITH SHIVA

This morning, instead of going to church, I take the scissors and cut off all the hair that remains on my head. There isn't much. Then I sweep up the poor tufts and strands from the bathroom floor and throw them in the wastebasket. I have been gathering my nerve toward this destruction for days; still it's difficult to actually pick up the scissors and snip. But it is also freeing. No more long, glittering strands on clothing and floors. No more wet wads to pick out of drains. Still, it isn't easy to sacrifice—to destroy—something as precious and intimate as your own hair.

Freedom, as Janis Joplin reminded us, is "just another word for nothing left to lose." With no hair left to lose, I did feel free.

"I am dancing with Shiva," I whisper as the last snip falls from behind my ear.

In the trinity of Hindu gods, Shiva fills an important role; he is known as the destroyer and he balances the functions of Vishnu, the preserver of the universe and Brahma, the supreme, eternal deity. When the Ganges overflows, taking with it crops and cattle and sometimes entire families, it is the work of Shiva—the purger, the scourer.

How can such a destructive force be worshipped?

Hindus understand that there can't be new creation without destruction of the old order. And this concept is not really alien in the West either, for Christianity asserts that you must "die to the old" in order to realize rebirth—resurrection. And while destruction may be painful, it can clear the way for joy.

Still, when you are dancing with Shiva—as I am in this experience of alopecia—you are caught in the vortex of destruction and the promise of new creation requires a faith that is very strong indeed. As the hair from my head spills down my shoulders and onto the floor, I feel very much in the clutch of destruction and I'm not sure my faith is strong enough.

Still, I am trying to embrace this new dancing partner who comes to me adorned with snakes and smeared with the ashes of the crematoria. His dance is the cosmic dance. The energy of it generates and sustains creation. His snakes, which are able to regenerate the skins they shed, remind me that my hair will regenerate. The deer that are sometimes depicted with Shiva, are able to re-grow the antlers they seasonally lose. And when Shiva's monsoons finally end, India's valleys transform from desert into verdant and fertile farmlands.

The seasonal monsoons offer me a new thought: this is an appropriate time of year to be shorn of my hair. The outdoors is frozen and scoured, shriven of plants. My head is shriven. Lent, in my language of Christianity, is approaching.

So whirl me faster, Shiva, god of destruction. Dance me toward transformation.

500 HATS

In *The 500 Hats of Bartholomew Cubbins*, a popular Dr. Seuss book, a little boy named Bartholomew has five hundred hats. I have discovered a Web site that has that many and more. For someone with alopecia areata or a chemotherapy-induced case of baldness, Headcovers.com is as wonderful as the tale of Bartholomew Cubbins.

In the story, King Derwin marches by a group of townspeople and with his neighbors, the little boy named Bartholomew respectfully removes his hat. But when he does, another hat appears. King Derwin's irritation with the child grows into fury as one hat after another—each fancier than the one before—keeps sprouting on the boy's head. But when the five-hundredth hat appears, King Derwin is so dazzled, he offers to buy it for five hundred gold pieces.

Visiting the Headcovers.com site, I feel like King Derwin. Each hat offered on the site seems more wonderful than the one before it, and each promises full head coverage. No more reason to worry about peepholes to my baldness that come along with the adjustable bands on the backs of traditional baseball caps.

Turbans and wraps, caps and fancy hats, scarves and hats with fringes of hair around the edges—Headcovers.com is a treasure trove for the bald.

My hat order comes to more than a hundred dollars. If I don't grow hair soon, I'll own more hats myself than Bartholomew Cubbins.

HAIR ABUSE

Maybe I was destined for alopecia. Maybe it's just one more episode in the sad biography of my hair. Early on I got my first clue that something was wrong with me—and what was wrong about me was my hair.

"How could you let them *do-o-o-o* that to her?"

My mother is clearly upset. I am three-years-old and am deeply involved with a butterscotch lollipop. My father and I have just returned from a trip to his barber—a trip that surely wasn't a unilateral decision on his part. There was a high chair, a crisp blue and white striped sheet, and afterward a basket full of lollipops.

"Do you want cherry?" the barber asks encouragingly. "Root beer? Butterscotch?"

Butterscotch. What a heavenly word! I am enchanted.

"Butterscotch, please," I whisper.

Now, savoring the butterscotch, I understand that something has gone wrong, something having to do with my hair. I'd been taken to the barber shop because my mother was unhappy with my hair. Now my hair is short and I have a butterscotch lollipop and my mother is still unhappy. One incidence of dissatisfaction with my hair has just been traded for another.

Attempts to improve me by improving my hair continue. Aunt Mary joins the effort. She and my mother discuss my hair over the phone. Aunt Mary has found someone on the West Side who is a genius—an absolute genius. Until my mother tires of the trek across town every time my thick, fast-growing hair needs cutting—and until it is determined that the results aren't worth it anyway—I am driven to the West Side every couple of weeks to be shorn by Louie the Genius. The genius has bad breath. I cringe when he blows hairs off my neck.

I notice that my sister isn't subjected to the same hair ordeals I am made to endure. Grandma capably weaves Meg's hair into two blonde braids each morning and everyone leaves her alone. I get the message that Meg cannot be improved upon. She is perfect, whereas perfection, in my case, hasn't yet been achieved and from all the fuss that is continually kicking up, I realize it isn't likely to be. My imperfection, manifested by my hair, is a sore point for all.

My father sends me from the dinner table to secure a curtain of hair that keeps falling over one eye.

"Who do you think you are?" he asks. "Veronica Lake?"

How could I think I was Veronica Lake?

I don't even know who Veronica Lake is.

Aunt Mary thinks a Toni Home Permanent would help. I am driven to the West Side again where Aunt Mary's guestroom has been transformed into a hair salon. The Toni Home Permanent is more awful that anything I've ever experienced. My hair is soaked with a foul solution, then small bits of it are wrapped in squares of tissue, rolled onto tiny pink plastic chicken bones and daubed with a suffocating substance called neutralizer. The neutralizer makes my nose run and would make my eyes water except I am already crying as I hunch over Aunt Mary's dressing table with neutralizer dripping down my neck and running under my collar.

Scolding is apparently my mother's role in the perm processes. I am told to sit up straight, to stop that sniffing, and for goodness sakes, to be grateful for all that is being done on my behalf.

When the permed hair is finally revealed, my tears morph into loud sobs. Great clouds of frizz spring from my head. I look like a giant scouring pad.

The perm grows out, but they come at me again. I am taken back to Aunt Mary's salon for Round Two. One good thing comes out of Round Two, and for it, I will always be grateful to my sister.

While Aunt Mary and my mother are working on me (Aunt Mary soaking, winding and dabbing and my mother scolding and exhorting), Meg applies neutralizer-soaked cotton pads to each of the four posts of Aunt Mary's mahogany guestroom bed. She pats each pad down efficiently, chemically removing the elegant finish. Four white scars forever testify to the Toni Home Permanent experience and to Meg's selfless act of counter-terrorism.

To prepare for Easter Sunday, that day of hats and best dresses, my mother ties my hair up in strips of torn sheets. I look like Topsy. The next morning my released hair protrudes from under my straw Breton in odd fits and starts, riotous curls alternating with straight hanks where the curl "didn't take".

The sight of my hair as I sit at the dinner table annoys my father. Then a good idea strikes him.

"I'll cut it," he declares. On the spot he attacks my hair with the desk shears. He is not careful and chunks of the thick stuff rain around my shoulders. He hacks it short as a boy's. Then he produces a bottle of gluey hair tonic, shakes a liberal dollop onto my head and massages it in. My head rocks back and forth as if whiplashed and tears spring to my eyes, but the hair, shellacked to my scalp, stays out of my eyes.

By junior high, I am the one abusing my hair. Bobby pins are the first instruments of torture. I am careful to wash my hair each night so it will be fresh and bouncy the next day. Then, following the diagrams in *American Girl* and *Seventeen*, I twirl bits of hair into snails and skewer each perfect circle with two crisscrossed bobby pins. With a turban created from a silk scarf, I try to sleep on this creation. My hair is often still wet the next morning and all that bobby pinning amounts to nothing as damp strands draggled down in a very un-*American Girl* way.

Brush rollers have a real patch on bobby pins. No more bobby pin marks—just smooth waves. But sleeping on brush rollers is quite painful until you get used to it. After a while, I seem to develop ridges in my scalp and the rollers are easier to sleep on.

In my thirties I continue the hair abuse, this time with Clairol shampoo-in color. I choose a shade as near my natural one as possible, aiming just to brighten the flat dead-mouse color nature has dealt me. But after years of perking up with Clairol, I forget what my natural color actually looks like.

Once at a party, a man who ran a ritzy Newbury Street hair salon reached over and gathered a bunch of my hair in his fist.

"What I wouldn't give," he said passionately, "to get my hands on this! A nice layered cut, I think! With this hair," he rhapsodized, "I could do such wonders!"

As tactfully as I could, I disentangled my hair from his grip and sloped my shoulder out from under his forearm. Beside me I could feel Don bristle and prepare to growl. With vague promises, I gently side-stepped his offer to visit his salon. Any hair salon, but especially one on toney Newbury Street, fills me with horror and anxiety. They say that public speaking is the number one fear among people. I don't mind public speaking, but please don't throw me into a hair salon.

And now this—alopecia areata. One more event in my hair history. And I can be pretty sure the final chapter isn't written yet. Or is it?

ADJUSTING THE MEDS

Dr. Chapin's nurse is horrified by my scalp scabs. I assure her that my head is supposed to look this way, and I recite: "Irritation causes hair to grow."

She backs out of the examining room looking dubious.

Dr. Chapin seems unfazed by the site of my glowing, infected head, but she snatches up a magnifying glass for a closer look. She pronounces that some new hair is growing. Then she adjusts my meds.

She retires the tretinoin cream (a.k.a. Retin A a.k.a. tar) temporarily.

She retires the anthralin cream temporarily.

I'm not sorry to see either of them go.

I am to continue using Rogaine for Women *but only on the left side.* This is for experimental purposes to see if the left side will grow faster than the right. (Or to see if any hair grows at all, I think sarcastically.)

I am to start a course of antibiotics—Zithromax—in preparation for a scalp biopsy. Ah ha! I conclude that

Dr. Chapin is more concerned about this irritated scalp than she lets on. Infection has trumped irritation. We've gone too far.

NEEDLES

In tandem with the scalp biopsy, Dr. Chapin plans to launch a course of cortisone injections in my scalp at the end of February. Like the topical medications I have been faithfully using, the cortisone is supposed to stimulate hair growth, but it is reputed to be a more aggressive stimulant than the topicals.

Dr. Chapin explains that a shot of cortisone can excite sleeping hair follicles and will, almost certainly, cause hair to grow.

This is elating news!

She explains that it will sometimes jumpstart hair all over the head and sometimes will only initiate hair at the injection site. She also says that the hair may not be permanent.

But I am excited—eager for the needle therapy to begin and optimistic that in my case, hair will happen. I can't imagine not having a thick mane of hair.

In preparation for three needles in the head—two for the cortisone and one for the biopsy—Dr. Chapin prescribes a topical anesthetic, which I am to apply two hours before my appointment in her office. Since I routinely wait an hour before she makes her appearance, I wonder if I am meant to apply the anesthetic just one hour before the time written on my appointment card. But I decide that a question like this would sound too impertinent so I keep quiet and nod like the dutiful patient who follows every directive to the letter.

Three spots on my head are marked for the needles: one site at the back where the red, burned reaction is the most severe will be the biopsy site; then an area on each temple is designated for the cortisone injections. For the sake of balance, in case the hair jumpstart is successful, Dr. Chapin warns me to balance the shot sites.

But needles are needles, right? And what harm can a few more do? So while I am waiting for the biopsy/ injection appointment to come up, I make an appointment with an acupuncturist.

The idea is inadvertently suggested by a fellow martial arts student.

"I am seeing an acupuncturist," he tells me as we sit sat side by side clacking our chopsticks at a Chinese New Year banquet.

"*I've* been looking for an acupuncturist!" I tell him, discovering that it is true. "But I don't want to go to just anyone, and I don't know who is really good."

My companion successfully secures a piece of duck with his chopsticks and explains that our martial arts instructor recommended a therapist with the decidedly un-Oriental name of Martin Kelly.

So before Dr. Chapin takes up her needlework, I make an appointment for a free acupuncture consultation.

Martin Kelly, who suggests I call him Kell, seems to run his business with very little overhead. He answers his own phone and makes his own appointments. Payments, I read in the terms posted on his waiting room wall, are preferably cash at the time of patient visits and insurance reimbursements are the entire responsibility of the patient.

Kell's offices are light and bright. George Winston's piano music leaks pleasantly through the clean, white rooms and a handsomely-framed print of bamboo fills one wall. It is, I decide, a comfortable place to be.

The free consultation takes about twenty minutes. I do most of the talking and Kell does all of the note writing. Finally I wind down. "Do you think acupuncture could help?"

He looks at me squarely and I like his failure to make hurried promises. "I suggest you try it for six or eight sessions and see what happens. In the meantime, I want to do some studying about this. While I have treated hair loss before, I've never worked with anything as extreme as yours."

In Chinese medicine, Kell explains, issues with skin, hair, and nails are associated with the kidneys and he suggests there may be some imbalances in my blood that need correction.

This makes sense to me, and I tell him I'd like to try six sessions. In preparation, Kell gives me a seven page health history questionnaire to complete before my first visit. I have homework, and so does he. We both have responsibilities in this treatment. That's good. As a contexturalist—one who believes you can only understand things in context with other things—I appreciate his holistic approach.

Then, in an odd shift of attitude and emphasis, I offer a confession: "I know my hair is going to grow back. It is going to grow back whether I apply all those topical medications Dr. Chapin has prescribed or whether I don't. I know it will grow back whether we do acupuncture or not. I know all this. But even with this conviction and the sense that regrowth is starting even now, I am careful about applications, I intend to go ahead with the cortisone treatment, and I am eager to start acupuncture. And I don't understand all this."

Kell nods.

And I leave his office, carefully carrying my questionnaire.

OTHER PEOPLE'S PITY

Sometimes a certain look comes over the face of the person I'm in conversation with, and I know what's coming. She or he is going to ask about the progress of my disease. The inquiry is always framed the same way—in a way the speaker thinks of as positive and optimistic.

"Well, how's the hair coming?" (The hearty approach.)

"Any new hair growing yet?" (The cautiously hopeful tack.)

And of course the dreaded and ubiquitous "What are they doing about it?

They. The unnamed medical gurus who are responsible for healing and correcting all things. *They* are clearly not doing their jobs here.

I am discovering that the same people are making the same inquiries—sometimes on a weekly basis. I know they are wishing the best for me and I know that they are disappointed on my behalf. But how much explaining can I do to someone to whom I've already explained it all?

The folks wearing the looks of unqualified pity seem completely unaware of their expressions. When I see these expressions, I feel called on to counterbalance their horror with a load of good cheer. I notice that I'm starting to adopt an upbeat and optimistic countenance that is bordering on the bubbly, possibly even the giddy. But in my mind's eye I see invisible cartoon bubbles above their heads, each containing the words: "Thank God this isn't happening to me!"

Well, it *is* happening to me, I want to say crisply, "and I'll tell you something—it isn't as bad as you seem to think. I'm still who I've always been. Please try to see past my head and help me remember who I am."

I can't stand pity! Do anything, but don't feel sorry for me!

SPARKING THE CHI

Kell has determined a course of acupuncture treatment. Hair, in Chinese medicine, is considered the province of the blood and by association, the kidneys. He will use the needles to tone the blood, nourish the yin chi and bring the yang chi to my skull in order to stimulate the sleeping hair follicles.

Each session has two twenty-minute treatments. For the first round, I lie on my back gazing at the places where the walls join the ceiling. Then I close my eyes as Kell inserts the needles, one by one, along my hairline. A single needle zings into the top of my head. A needle goes into each of my wrists and then into each of my ankles. And finally, a single needle is inserted in the dantien, the spot several inches below my navel.

As a student of tai chi chuan, I am familiar with the dantien, and it makes sense to me that a needle would be placed there in the storehouse of energy—what the Chinese call "chi" or "qi." When I began a Pilates course, I was pleased to encounter a similar recognition of the power of the dantien. In Pilates terminology the band of muscles that encircles the body just south of the beltline is called the "powerhouse," and the Pilates exercises focus on strengthening this core.

Everything is connected. Nothing can be seen in isolation.

Wednesday is a good day for chi.

In my acupuncture session, Kell is quietly plonging needles into my skull.

"Is that one going into the crown chakra?" I ask.

"Exactly so. It is to draw energy up into your head."

Kell continues traveling south, inserting needles into my wrists, abdomen and feet. He focuses a gentle heat lamp on my belly, dims the lights and withdraws, saying, "Now your job is to rest."

I lie peacefully, and in a few minutes, begin to watch the colors that materialize on the insides of my eyelids. Deep rose fades to pale gray then swims back again to rose, rich and vibrant, turning into paler shades as if someone had turned a sweater inside out. The rose colors mutate into peach tones ... subside. And so nearly twenty minutes pass.

Suddenly I have the impression of an overwhelming, but not unpleasant, warmth flooding my head. The heat lasts perhaps a minute, not much more.

Preceded by a gentle rap, Kell enters the room and begins harvesting the needles from my ankles, working up. When he arrives at my head, I mention the sensation to him.

He smiled. "That's the good yang chi. It's working."

We are both encouraged.

In my internal martial arts class we are beginning to study hsing yi chuan. Known as shape-mind boxing, hsing yi is a cousin of the better known tai chi, but instead of tai chi's steady, gentle movements, this form demands that the practitioner gather internal energy then release it briefly and explosively before returning to soft (yin) chi. At the end of the class our coach cautions us. "Too much energy can go to the head. People sometimes get migraines from practicing this, so pace yourselves."

My energy has certainly been stirred, and I am delighted to hear his caution. One more way to bring good yang chi to my wounded head.

At home, Don is on the sofa watching a TV show about submarines. I curl in beside him and he begins massaging my bald dome. He has good hands. Strong hands. Dogs crave his attention for he seems to know just how to touch them. His sympathetic fingers and palms work on my head. Afterward my head practically glows with warmth. I hurry into the kitchen and catch up with him by the sink.

"Feel!" I command.

"Your head's hot," he exclaims. "Really hot to the touch."

I am triumphant. Three good chi surges in one day. I can almost feel the hair begin to bloom.

MORE NEEDLES

Dr. Chapin is examining the two quarter-sized patches of thick, dark hair that are the results of her cortisone shots in my scalp. As hoped, the shots four weeks ago have stimulated some growth, but the greater hope—that they would encourage full-head coverage—is sadly unrealized.

"Do you mind the dents the shots caused?" she wants to know.

Dents? I hadn't noticed the dents. But sure enough, there they are. Still surprised, I say that no, I don't mind them, but later curiosity sends me Googling again. Sure enough, there they are on one of the alopecia sites. Their technical name is dells, and now that they've been called to my attention, they begin to look very prominent.

"Well then," she says briskly having heard that I don't mind the dents, "why don't we try a few more shots? Say six?"

I agree that six sounds good, but rather than plunge ahead right in her office and take the shots without anesthetic, I opt to mark my own target spots. If I'm going to grow new hair, I want to design it myself.

For this project, I enlist my dear husband's help. He is, after all, an artist and who would be better to draft the hair targets?

"I want the shots in the baldest spots," I direct, "but I also want them symmetrical, you know?"

Don wields an eyebrow pencil and draws bold circles, which I fill in a few hours later with the numbing linocane. Since I don't want the pencil lines or the anesthetic to rub off, I carefully press a sheet of clear plastic food wrap over my dome, then gingerly pull my newsboy's cap over the plastic wrap. I feel like a deviled egg being prepared for transport to a picnic.

Dr. Chapin obligingly sinks her needles into the spots of choice. "I'll use just a little more than usual," she says, pushing a plunger and seeming to rotate it slightly. "We're going to give this every chance."

TEMPORARY HAIR

"You could always get a wig." Dr. Chapin offers this parting counsel as she leaves the examining room.

"But I have a wig," I protest. "I just don't like it."

Dr. Chapin pulls her eyebrows up toward her hairline, smiles and explains, as if to a rather slow child, "Then get another one." And—swish—she is gone.

I have permission, and it is all so simple. I can own more than one wig! Like Dorothy in Oz who could have gone home all along, it has always been in my power to have more than one wig. I just needed to be told by some great and powerful wizard that it was alright.

And who says I have to get a wig that mimics my old hair? Time to break out of the mold. Time to have a hairstyle with a personality that isn't like the one that I've been living with all these years. My alopecia has suddenly given me permission to try something new—to *be* somebody new.

But I'm damned if I'll go back to Humberto! I go to the Web instead.

The very next morning I spend an hour on the Headcovers site shopping for a wig. Instead of copying my old hair, as Humberto and I had tried to do with the pageboy bob, I look for something different. I want something short. Something ... well, kicky.

After some blundering about, I eventually find a tape measure, pass it around my skull, and following Headcovers' directions, discover that I must shop in their petite section unless I want to risk losing my hair in traffic or high wind. The selection in the petite section isn't quite as broad, but never mind. It is adequate for my needs, and I eventually choose a short "do" that will expose my ears and put pixie bangs across my forehead.

Then there's the matter of color. Even with the color swatches provided and the best of descriptive copywriting, making a color selection is a bit like buying a lottery ticket— you can't know if you are picking a winner. So I select something that I hope is ash blonde and key in my order.

The Giver-of-Permission Voice speaks again: "You know, if the color is wrong or you don't like the style, *you can always order another one!*"

And so a petite wig named Josie is on her way to me within minutes. Because I am suddenly in a rush, I spring for overnight delivery. On a cold, cold day, the deliveryman brings Josie right to my door.

I try the wig on and am astonished to see an uncanny resemblance to my sister Meg. The new hair has silvery highlights. It looks casual and elegant at the same time. I think I look good. No, I think I look great!

Josie and I, however, throw Don completely off balance when he comes home from work.

"Please, he says, "just please tell me before you spring one of these new looks on me. One day you're bald, the next day you're wearing a hat. And then there you are in hair I've never seen before. I need a little time to adjust to who my wife is going to be each evening."

The request seems reasonable. I promise to give notice.

Getting up the nerve to go out in public with Josie takes a little time. We choose to make our debut at a memorial service simply because that's the first opportunity that comes along. Don and I and Josie take a pew in the back of the church where I hope we will escape notice. But like many of the best laid plans, this one goes "agly" at the end of the service when the funeral director asks those in the very last pew to go down the center aisle to greet the bereaved family. Don and I are the third pew sent forward on this mission. I tramp self-consciously down the center aisle and bend to grasp George's hand, hoping he will at least recognize me with Josie sitting on my head smug as a cat on a cushion. He does! Doesn't even do a double take. What relief! I pass along the pew of mourners murmuring platitudes of condolence and escape up the side aisle feeling the eyes of the congregation upon me.

At the collation following the service, people nearly sprain ankles getting over to me to compliment me on my new haircut. I make an important decision in real time.

"It's a wig," I say frankly. "All of my hair has fallen out."

This announcement is invariably followed by expressions of surprise, shock, and sympathy

"Why are you telling everyone that?" Don hisses into my ear. He is speaking without moving his lips.

"Because," I reply, "they are going to see me sometimes with just a cap or a kerchief, and eventually they will see me with a buzz cut that is growing out. I think it's better to be up-front right at the start and avoid questions later."

He shrugs. It makes a certain kind of sense.

But as Josie and I continue to make occasional public appearances—and I limit my Josie-wearing to meetings, public events, and any speeches I might make—

a new issue begins to dawn on me. How bad had my hair looked before alopecia?

When I eventually start leaving Josie at home, will the compliments drop away? Or will people ask me when was I going to return to that nice hair style I'd had last winter?

"You'll have to take the wig to the hair dresser and have them style your hair to match it," suggests my friend Mary.

This is a good point. I make a mental note to do that and imagine myself laughing away with a hairdresser who is trying to shape and color my new crop of hair into a clone of Josie.

"This is temporary hair," I tell the fellow who holds the bank door open for me and who has just complemented Josie as he gallantly ushers me inside. "But it turns out," I add ruefully, "that the other hair was temporary, too."

HEY! SHE'S GOT MY HAIR!

Sometimes I catch a glimpse of my hair—my *old* hair—my hair the way it used to look (or maybe the way I wanted it to look). And this hair will be on the head of a woman marching along a sidewalk or bending over the grapefruit in the supermarket's produce section. Then I experience a spasm of recognition followed with a clutch of real longing, that stops me in my tracks to stare or pulls my foot off the accelerator while I visually follow the hair robber as she goes on her way.

I remember. And I grieve for a moment for the hair that once was and for the present loss.

I think this reaction must be like the loss of a loved family member. Even when you think you've accepted the unalterable fact of the situation—the reality—something happens to jog the elbow of memory and for a second or two you forget.

SISTERS UNDER THE SCARF

The Colonel's lady and Judy O'Grady are sisters under the skin. Rudyard Kipling

"Do you have what I have?" the woman demands.

It is Joanne M. and she is standing right in front of me, staring. I know her only slightly, but I *do* know she is being treated for breast cancer.

I am suddenly reminded that my clever newsboy's cap can't fully hide my shiny sidewalls. So much for disguise.

I smile a little ruefully. "I guess not. I've lost my hair because of alopecia."

She gives my head another appraising scan before she sweeps away.

While sudden hair loss produces many issues that are common to people experiencing both chemotherapy and alopecia, there are some significant differences.

"I knew what was going to happen," says Lauren, now fully recovered from her bout with breast cancer, "so when my hair started coming out, I just shaved the rest off."

Joanne M. echoed that experience. "They told me that next week I would start losing my hair. Well, I didn't want to mess around with it falling out one hair at a time, so I just cut every single bit off." She assumes a triumphant look.

Chemotherapy does offer a road map of sorts: you are going to lose your hair and you understand why. You also know your hair will grow back. I don't have the luxury, if you want to call it that, of that road map. So, unlike Lauren and Joanne and some others, I didn't immediately shave off my remaining hair. Instead, I kept hoping the deciduation would stop. That day never came.

For the person with alopecia areata or some other idiopathic problem, hair loss is a sneak attack. There has been no preparation for the condition and acceptance may be weeks or months or even forever away. It takes time to understand what is happening and even longer to accept it.

Moreover, there is no guarantee that the Alopecian is going to get new hair; there are only some dismal percentages and rules-of-thumb. The younger you are when hair loss occurs, the less chance you have of seeing it regenerate. (At least my advanced age was working in my favor here.) If you have hair loss over the entire body (universalis) or if you lose all your hair (totalis), your chances of regrowth are lessened. And if your fingernails exhibit a characteristic stippling, as if pinpricked in neat rows, that's one more strike against you.

People I've spoke to about chemo-induced hair loss usually explain that the hair started to grow back as soon as the chemotherapy ended. And it grew back evenly.

A cancer patient has to deal with issues far more serious than baldness. Compared to the life-threatening risks that cancer poses, hair loss is easy. The Alopecian may have the "luxury" of focusing completely on the hair loss situation; for alopecia—frightening and unpleasant though it may be—is not life threatening.

The patient having chemo may feel physically ill or lethargic—a dispiriting state of health, to say the least. The Alopeciac probably feels physically fine—I certainly do. Neither my energy nor my appetite has flagged.

A person being treated with chemo can probably count on having a support group of other patients and survivors who have been there ahead of her. These sisters can act as consultants and guides through the experience.

Unless the alopecia sufferer can turn to a cancer survivor who has experienced hair loss, a support system may be largely unavailable. On the other hand, I began to discover a vast sorority out there. While I never did meet anyone else who had directly suffered from alopecia areata, I knew lots of people who had experienced hair loss from chemotherapy, and they were generous to me in the sharing of tips and tricks for coping with sudden baldness. But encouragement and optimism is the best thing that they all offer. And there hasn't been a soul who hasn't held out hope. They say: "Of course your hair will grow back. And it usually grows back better than ever."

Thank you, sisters.

BEANHEAD

It's a genetic thing: a few of us in my family have been born with smaller than normal heads. Oh, not a big deal, just a little smaller and sort of pointy. Beanheads, we call ourselves jokingly. We try on each other's hats and hoot with laughter as the hats for normal sized heads fall down about our ears or balance on our eyeglass frames. My niece Molly, one of my very favorite beanheads, got herself fitted with a child's bicycle helmet and insisted I try it. It fit perfectly and we laughed till we could hardly stand.

There is rarely more than one beanhead in a generation. My mother was one. I am one. Molly makes three, although there are still children to be born in the next generation and the possibility for another beanhead is always present.

When I lost my hair, my beanhead became cruelly exposed. There was to be no more hiding under teased hair. Beanheaded *and* bald. As if there needed to be more proof that life is unfair.

THE ILLUSTRATED EYEBROW

Appreciate your eyebrows! They are the gutters of the face. They sop up unpleasant substances like shampoo and sweat. They give character and personality and erase the "Vacancy" sign that the naked face hangs out.

Before alopecia, I had looked upon eyebrows simply as a beauty issue—as just another hair detail to be plucked, shaped and penciled in. My main eyebrow issue was choosing a pencil that matched my hair color.

Alopecia areata erased my eyebrows and eyelashes, along with my other body hair, causing me to be constantly startled and re-startled by the bald look of my face. Without eyebrows, I look tired. Anemic. Expressionless. Some days I think I look insane.

Working from memory, I begin drawing my eyebrows on every morning.

This is more difficult than it sounds.

I found I could sketch the right one without too much trouble, but illustrating a matching left brow is a challenge that seems beyond my skill. I didn't notice my amateur drawing right away, and I'm afraid I went out in the world on several occasions with a left brow half an inch higher that it's cousin on the right. Have you ever had a conversation with someone who is wearing mismatched earrings? It is disconcerting. Your eyes dart from the left ear to the right and back again. My eyebrows must have produced the same unsettled affect in people. I began laboring over my illustrative chore.

I grouse about my difficulty to my husband.

"Well, of course you can't get your eyebrows even," he says matter-of-factly. "Your eyes aren't the same, didn't you know that? One is higher than the other."

So here's one more fact to add to my private inventory of physical flaws. No, I had not known that.

"Everybody—most everybody anyway—has uneven eyes," Donald went on. "It isn't just you."

As a lifelong artist and sometime portrait painter, Don has made a career of studying people, so I believe him.

But it doesn't help my dilemma of getting eyebrows onto my face.

I found out you can buy false eyebrows. Did you know that? I had known about false eyelashes, of course, but I've never dreamed anyone would buy false eyebrows! I made the eyebrow discovery while I was shopping for wigs online, and for a while I considered ordering a pair. For thirty-five dollars, plus shipping, I could eliminate my problem of drawing freehand brows. But as with all things, false eyebrows come with their own encyclopedia of difficulties. Removing the eyebrow adhesive is one challenge. And another issue is shaping the brows once you've bought them. Apparently they are a one-size-fits-all deal. The brows arrive as a straight set of hairs arranged on a backing, and during the application, you are supposed to determine the arch or slant you desire. I figure this would just be a variation on my present problem of drawing a matched set. I can see myself gluing on a pair of brows, then finding that one was considerably out of kilter— positioned too close to the bridge of my nose while its mate was stationed far west of its target.

With a small sigh, I pass up the false eyebrow opportunity. Still, it's nice to know that you can buy a pair if you want them.

GOING TURTLE

*Consider the turtle; he makes progress only when he
sticks his neck out. Anon.*

I have a multi-color down on my head, concentrated mostly
in the center of my scalp like an erratic Mohawk. I know it
isn't pretty but I am stubbornly pleased with it for some
reason and decide to venture out in semi-public with this
semi-naked head. When I make this decision, the gender
gap gaps.

Women, as a class, are interested, curious,
applauding, encouraging, questioning, and generally
delighted. They want to touch my head, want to feel the
short stubs sprouting there. They walk three-hundred-sixty
degree circles around me to inspect my head from all sides.
They inquire about the color and offer opinions garnered
from their own experiences and observations.

Men seem embarrassed. Most avert their eyes or
behave as if there were nothing at all unusual about my

head, and if they just don't call attention to my obvious baldness, maybe I won't notice it either. Maybe it just won't *be*.

So I choose my episodes of exposure carefully.

My sister is the first—and safest—person to whom I feel comfortable revealing my hairless squash. I stick my bald dome out the door as her car rolls in, and she crows in delight to see the peach down on my skull.

"That's just what Candy's hair looked like when it started coming in!"

The minister, invited to dinner, is the next guest to have to endure a bald hostess. I figure in his line of work, he's seen just about everything anyway, and this won't be a big deal. And it isn't. But for the first time, I notice the true male pattern of tact; he refrains from mentioning any subject north of my shoulders. To clear the air, I finally bring the subject up myself, and then we are able to chat our way through a very pleasant evening, just as though I were a normal person.

I would have preferred to undertake the head version of going turtle when I had an even growth of new hair. But we don't always get our druthers, and I've gotten tired of waiting. So now that I've produced a motley strip of hair down the center of my skull, I feel ready to start taking off my cap. The sidewalls, as Don calls my temples, are still glossy and bare, but if I can get used to the look of my own head, I figure other people, who have so much less invested, have to be able to take it.

Oddly, it is around strangers that going turtle is the hardest. A simple errand like going to the supermarket requires careful hatting. How funny that the opinions and judgments of strangers seem to matter more than those of family and friends.

I observe that the more comfortable I appear to be with my own alopecia areata, the more comfortable those around me seem to feel. But I notice that people, who are not completely comfortable within their own skins, never seem to gain a sense of comfort around me.

I discover that when I don't offer a preamble that calls attention to my head, people seem reluctant to introduce the subject of my baldness; but if I call attention to my head as I doff my cap, then folks are open to comment and seem to feel more comfortable.

DORMANCY

Cold. My boots make *unch-unch-unch* sounds on the rims
of crusted snow and on the frozen grass. The sun, this
early March morning, is bright but there is no heat in it.
My bald head within its shroud of a woolen cap and a polar
fleece head sock is reasonably warm. The dog idles from
bush to grass tuffet sniffing and reading stories of animals
that have passed. Waiting while she reads, I stand there
examining the bare branches of my neighbor's weeping
mulberry tree, remembering the hot afternoon we planted
it last summer.

We'd gone—Patty, Steve, and I—one hot day to the
nursery to look for flowering trees. They found the
mulberry and I'd chosen a Japanese snowbell. The sun had
been brutal that day and I'd worn a straw hat to protect the
hair I didn't know I'd soon lose.

The mulberry branches are at my eye level and I
am surprised to see the tree is covered with tiny, tight

buds—a promise, on this cold morning, that spring will arrive and new growth will indeed come out of these dead-looking twigs. I eagerly look for other signs of stirring dormancy. The lilacs have fat pale green buds, even though the temperature is far below freezing. And hurrying home at last to the warmth of my kitchen, I stop to interview the snowbell and am encouraged to find that it too seems to have survived the winter and is showing vestigial buds.

Continuing toward the kitchen, I think about my dormant head. Is there vestigial hair in there? Just waiting for warmer, longer days to germinate? Waiting for the long, cold winter to end?

SPRING

BALD AS A BEAN

CHIA PET

"You are beginning to look like a Chia pet," Don remarks.

"Like a what?"

"You know, one of those ceramic animals—a dog or a pig—that they pour water on and it grows grass that's supposed to look like hair. That green, spikey, sticking-up-sort of grass."

There is indeed a crown of light brown hair on the very top of my head. Dr. Chapin uses a magnifying glass to examine it.

"There is even some new hair growing," she exclaims triumphantly. "See here, fine, light hairs just up here."

She guides my fingers to the spot and indeed, rubbing my hand lightly, just micro-inches from the skull, I feel the beginnings of soft, new hair. It feels the way I'd imagine the velvety new growth on a deer's antler to feel.

I proudly display my velvet to Don—tangible proof that hair is growing back at last. The down on my head is like newly planted grass—frail, soft spikes that look vulnerable to the tramping footstep. Baby grass, I'd tell my children when they were small and were being instructed not to step on their father's newly seeded lawn.

"Shh-hh, the baby grass is growing. Don't disturb it."

The alopecia areata is reacting exactly according to The Seasons Theory. I remember to give special thanks for this triumph.

THE LEGEND OF THE BLACK-HAIRED MONK

He lost his way while traveling between two monasteries, or so the story goes, and for twenty years, this monk of western China wandered in the wilderness. The path he'd followed disappeared, seemed to reveal itself again, but ultimately vanished for good, and the monk blundered up one blind canyon after another. At last he gave up and accepted his situation. He spent his time wandering, meditating, and searching for sustenance. But the land in that part of China offered very little vegetation. The main thing that grew in abundance was *he shou wu*—the polygonum plant—known more commonly as knotgrass. After twenty years of wilderness existence, the monk's wanderings brought him to a village. And miraculously, it was the very village where he had been born. With wonder, he entered the street where he had played as a child. The villagers hurried from their houses to greet the visitor. They recognized the monk almost at once—and he recognized them. But there was something that astonished both visitor and villagers. The monk saw that all the playmates of his childhood were gray-haired, and his contemporaries stared in amazement, for the monk's hair was black as jet and as thick as a youth's.

He soon became known as the black-haired monk, and ever after in China, the root of polygonum, has been prized for its ability to keep hair dark and abundant. *He shou wu* became known as the herb of the black-haired monk.

"Would I like to try this herb?" Kell wants to know.

My hair was never black, and I didn't care whether it grew in dark or gray, but the promise of abundance was a promise I'd pursue.

Like the black-haired monk, I decide I am prepared to wander, meditate, accept my fate, and now to sample the offerings of *he shou wu.*

So ... sure. I'll try it.

Kell has two bottles ready at my next appointment.

The powder ground from the polygonum root is dark brown and smells rather like *dit da jow*, a Chinese bruise liniment I sometimes use, which is to say it smells sort of like soy sauce. A tiny plastic spoon comes with the herb, and I am to mix three spoonfuls of powder into warm water and consume this three times a day, avoiding food for an hour before and after taking *he shou wu.*

The first glassful of the stuff looks evil indeed, but the taste is surprisingly pleasant.

Don, who doesn't have a gray hair in his head, but who is always eager to believe the worst—in other words, he *expects* to have gray hair (if, indeed he has any hair at all)—is quite interested in the potion. I offer him a swig.

"Tempting," he says, then hesitates. "But no."

ORIENTAL MEDICINE

Kell begins each acupuncture session with a chat, an inspection of my tongue and a pulse reading. Each is an important diagnostic tool in oriental medicine. Kell wants to know what is happening in my life: a head cold, unusual activity or even inactivity, are all events that contribute to or detract from my general health, and so are to be monitored and evaluated. He jots notes as we talk.

I have never much liked sticking out my tongue and saying "ahhh." Kell, however, is inordinately interested in my tongue. Practitioners of oriental medicine gain a lot of information this way. A tongue that is overly yang might be bright red, while one that is yang deficient, in other words, too yin, might be pale and puffy, as mine evidently was one day.

"Have you been feeling tired?" Kell asks as I pull my tongue back into my mouth and arrange it.

"Well, I've had a cold," I explain defensively.

"That explains it," he nods. "Well, let's feel your pulse."

Someone trained in pulse diagnosis feels the pulses in both wrists simultaneously, and he uses three fingers on each hand to do so. This is a difficult skill to master and not all acupuncturists use pulse diagnosis. Each finger searches for information related to one of the major body areas. My pulses are strong except for the kidney area—or so Kell claims.

Treating alopecia with acupuncture is an act of faith. If I had shoulder or knee pain, a single acupuncture treatment might bring me immediate relief, but even if the acupuncture needles could zing my sleeping follicles awake, the resultant hair wouldn't be noticed for a month or more.

So I choose to take the success of acupuncture on faith, but I do find I look forward to the treatment sessions which are very different from the treatments of my dermatologist.

In Dr. Chapin's office, I am accustomed to waiting an hour or more, first in her reception room, flipping through back issues of magazines, then in one of the treatment cubicles which are much colder and where the magazine selection is limited. Dr. Chapin's nurse pays a brief visit to ask a few questions and make a few notes, and then leaves me to shiver with my magazine while more minutes tick by. Finally Dr. Chapin sweeps in, and five minutes later I find myself at a tall desk paying my bill and making another appointment.

In Kell's office, the timing is completely reversed. I never wait for treatment. Kell is careful to demand punctuality of his clients, and since he values his clients' time and respects his own process, he doesn't double or triple book. I am ushered into the treatment room immediately where I receive an hour or more of treatment time without any sense of being given the bum's rush.

Alopathic medicine versus the Oriental approach, I guess. Both have their place. I wouldn't want to give up either in my quest for hair.

SCALP WOUNDS

I'm treading more carefully on the path of irritation therapy now, unwilling to subject my scalp to another season of infection. I hope my last infectious experience taught me a lesson. This time I'm limiting my applications of the topicals to every other day. Even so, my scalp is beginning to take on that seared and angry look again. Before the burns can morph into vicious scabs, I put away the tretinoin cream and the Retin A. For one thing, the therapy is interfering with my program of going turtle. While it is one thing to appear in semi-public as a baldy, it is quite something else to go out with a diseased and contagious-looking scalp.

To Kell, however, I am willing to reveal my wretched head.

"Are you taking your herbs?" he asks after he has pretended not to be shocked.

I burble a defensive answer about the difficulty fitting the *he shou wu* into my busy schedule.

Kell's tone is mild and tinged with no discernible reproach as he explains that the herb is a tonic. "It's not like a course of antibiotic. It's not something you have to take religiously and consume every last pill in the bottle. The herbs will just tone your blood." He smiles forgivingly. "So take it when you can."

Then he gives me a direct look. "You've got to prioritize, you know. This is important."

Kell is trying a slightly different approach now. As he plugs in a new arrangement of needles, including one that seems to be in my third eye, I feel warmth flooding my skull. I use the acupuncture session to visualize— something I have found difficult to do since the alopecia diagnosis. I am determined to make visualization a part of my daily schedule. And I promise myself to do *he shou wu* as well.

For the first time, I'm feeling that my approaches to treating the alopecia are in conflict. Dr. Chapin's caustic irritation therapy seems designed to abuse my hair into regrowing, while Kell's treatment seems encouraging and nurturing.

A gentler, more self-loving treatment feels right to me at this point. Tone the blood with herbs and stimulate the chi. Nurture and visualize. This kinder, more positive course suddenly seems the preferred path. By trying to combine the two, have I been setting up opposing protocols?

It is the Lenten season. Twice now, I've stood in the midst of a singing congregation intoning, "O, sacred head now wounded..." I wonder what images the others are getting? I keep flashing on my own wounded bean.

THE TAO OF BALDNESS
Do not attempt to go around the Cross. Edgar Cayce

Somewhere between the horror of pulling that first soapy wad of wet hair off my head and the moment I could stare calmly at the image reflected in my mirror, I have begun to accept what is happening to me. Acceptance is a process though. It involves a refusal to mourn the lost hair as well as the refusal to yearn for whatever hair I might someday have. Acceptance is simply looking at my naked skull right in the moment and without judgment.

This is the first step. The next step is to embrace it.

If acceptance is saying: "I have lost all my hair," then step two is saying: "This is where I need to be, and I want to experience this as fully as possible."

I am beginning to call this the Tao of Baldness. When there is something unpleasant in your path, don't try to avoid it and don't attempt to detour around it. Rather, step into the situation, determined to experience it as fully as possible. The path to growth is the straight path.

Now I have to find the courage to do more than look calmly at my baldness; I have to find a way to affirm it. Don suddenly gives me that opportunity. Sitting beside me on the sofa, he asks if I will let him paint a portrait of my bald head.

"Sure."

Don seats me in the wicker armchair in his studio, and I fix my gaze on a watercolor block as he begins to clutter about with his brushes and paints.

Have you wondered what a portrait subject thinks about while sitting so still? I think about how much I want to let my eyes close. They are growing so heavy. I think how much I want to scratch my chin ... my nose ... my eyebrow. I think about my hopes for this portrait. I want it to show me "warts and all" as they say, but at the same time, I hope it will reveal a beautiful woman who just happens to be bald. In other words, *my* warts should be lovely ones. After an hour's sitting, I am allowed to rise and stretch my legs.

The portrait is appalling!

I look like a crone. I resemble Gertrude Stein. And how have I never noticed how much like my mother I look? The portrait is ghastly, but the most shaking thing is that it is true. It is a likeness.

So much for acceptance. Can I really embrace this?

Don is kind.

"It doesn't work," he says simply. "We can do another sitting later, or we can make a new start."

We make a new start.

The second attempt is to be a smaller painting and the background will not be dark, and, I hope therefore, it will be less depressing. This time I pose in three-quarter profile with my eyes downcast. As I sit this time, I wonder if the downcast gaze and lowered head will make my jaw line sag into great jowls.

Ah, vanity. It works its wiles on the bald and unbald alike.

The result this time is better. Still not beautiful, but I am coming to terms with the fact that I would not be beautiful even with hair. I look like a comfortable, middle-aged woman whose head happens to look like a boiled egg.

Don is still not satisfied.

On the third try he works in charcoal, and he turns my face away and focuses on the nape of my neck and the back of my skull. The result pleases us both. I feel I could have this portrait framed and could hang it in the house—a testament to a part of my life. A historical record.

"How could you *do-oo-oo* that?" wails my daughter, unknowingly echoing the words and tone I'd heard my mother say about my hair some sixty years earlier. She is standing in front of the portrait.

"I take it you don't like it?"

"Why didn't you pose in your wig? You look great in your wig!"

Liz continues to stare judgmentally. Clearly she can't accept this fact about me—this baldness—but I feel the portrait is an important part of my path to self-acceptance. How to explain that? Ah, who can explain the Tao of Baldness?

"The Tao that can be told is not the eternal Tao."

DISCOURAGEMENT

"We'll just even it up."

Don is explaining why he wants to cut my hair which seems to be growing in the patchy, mottled way typical of alopecia. My present vision for my hair isn't grand. I would be delighted with a close-cropped, but even, hairstyle similar to the summer cuts small boys get when school is over and baseball season is in full swing.

I hear Don's clippers give one deep buzz on the back of my head.

"Don't cut it too short," I suddenly beg.

There is a beat of silence.

"Too late," he says softly.

Don proceeds to buzz and trim. Then he pinches up the bits of hair that have fallen to the towel that drapes my shoulders. These he presents to me. I inspect them closely, marveling at the color and texture. Soft as duck down. Charcoal, white, and brown. To me they seem inexpressibly beautiful. I, who never saved a lock of baby hair or a prom corsage, find myself uncharacteristically storing these few, tender tufts in a plastic sandwich bag.

In the next days, I keep taking my emotional temperature. I discover I feel sad. I keep my head covered. I had been so happy to reveal my weird Mohawk hairstyle, but now I feel bald and vulnerable again.

The low-grade depression continues for most of the week.

"Why am I so blue?" I keep asking myself. It has to be more than the haircut. Perception, I finally decide is the reason. Before Don took up the clippers I had perceived that my hair was growing back. Post-haircut, I find this perception is destroyed.

Then insult climbs onto injury. One night, returning from martial arts class, I take off the little black baseball cap I wear and discover the inside of it is littered with light, fine hairs. And they are mine! Hard to believe! At first I think the dog has gotten my cap and when I truly identify their author, my heart races. The last of what I'd thought was my new growth, my tender Mohawk, has come away from my head and I am truly stone bald.

I'm more than blue now. I feel gray; my outlook is gray; I'm drab, and I discover I am deeply disappointed. Part of the loss I feel is for my tender chia-pet hair and for several days I pick through these feelings as you'd sort through a pint of blueberries that are slowly going west. I discover, in this emotion-sorting, that I have lost something more than my hair; I've lost my belief in my Seasons Theory. And therefore I have lost hope.

The Seasons Theory has proved false. I had told myself that since I started losing my hair in the fall (deciduation), it stood to reason that the hair would grow back in the spring (regeneration and renewal). Now it's April and the regeneration isn't happening. In fact, exactly when my hair should be regenerating, it is deciduating. The daffodils and crocus that are beginning to blossom right on seasonal target are personally insulting to me. They are blooming and I am left behind.

As an antidote to this mild depression, I do what women often do: I decide to go shopping. In my case, I shop on the internet and buy another wig—Tia—a companion, or alter ego, to Josie.

I scold myself: "Who are you to decide a schedule for alopecia? Who told you this disease would precisely follow the calendar? Life, my girl, isn't as neat and tidy as the lists and outlines you make in your notebooks."

And so here is Easter again. And with it the annual celebration of the resurrection. I attend services wearing Josie and notice that while my hair has not come to life, my spirits have. The depression has lifted somewhat.

This time I have the wit to realize the lifting is probably not permanent. Depression will surely revisit, but next time I might be better prepared.

I used to read a picture book to my children: Leo the Late-Bloomer by Robert Kraus. Leo is a baby lion who isn't developing according to the benchmarks set by other baby lions. Leo's father is worried, but Leo's mother tells the old man not to worry, that Leo will bloom in time. Better late than never, the father thinks. Even so, the father watches carefully for signs of blooming. But Leo doesn't bloom. Every night the father checks for blooming signs. Nothing happens. The father again questions the mother who counsels patience and tells him that a watched bloomer doesn't bloom. Leo's father stops watching—even when the trees bloomed, he wasn't watching. That was okay though because Leo still wasn't blooming. And then one day, in his own good time, Leo bloomed!

Patience is one of the lessons I derive from this half-forgotten children's story. Blooms happen in their own time. And even though the trees are starting to bloom—

the sugar maple on the front lawn and the Norway maple in the backyard—nothing is sprouting on my head. In its own good time the hair will bloom.

Patience.

SALON EQUESTRIAN

Dr. Chapin is disappointed in the result of the last six cortisone injections. Standing in front of her while she frowns at my head, I feel like a student who has turned in careless and uncompleted homework. She and I agree, however, to each go to our respective corners and work harder. She pledges to do further research to see if any new medical wrinkles have appeared among the treatments for alopecia areata. From me, she exacts a pledge to continue the tar therapies and the odious Psoriatec applications as well as Rogaine applications and scalp massage.

Acting dutifully on my pledge, I download some massage techniques from various Web sites, apply a little lubricating oil and spend ten minutes massaging with my finger tips.

Bah!

There has to be a better way. That is why I'm in the car today, driving to the Equestrian Shop over on Route

114. I want to buy a horse curry, and the Equestrian Shop has tack buckets full of them; I am sure that among the horse care equipment I will find the perfect massage tool. Inside the tack shop, I duck offers of help from the salespeople. What I am going to say? That I am looking for a head massager?

"No thank you," I carol sweetly. "If I can't find what I want, I'll speak up."

My search of the tack buckets is thorough, and just when I think I can't find what I'm seeking, there it is! A green, rubber two-sided article with soft nubs. Perfect for massaging a hairless head.

When I apply this thing to my head, I have one moment of discomfort while the rubber tips press down; then they bend and I am suddenly massaging in comfortable circles, bringing circulation to my scalp. Needles, topicals, shampoos, and now horse curries—what a ludicrous disease is alopecia areata!

THE DANAS

Katie's invitation, issued in a batch e-mail, is wonderfully economical: "New York this spring? How 'bout the last day of April till May 2?" In Florida, Michigan, Ohio, and Massachusetts, the summonsed DANAs respond. Within four days the dates are confirmed and flight numbers, flight times and cell phone numbers are being e-mailed through cyberspace.

The DANAS are preparing to convene. If you could return for one night to 1959, you'd see a living room full of sixteen-year-old girls—girls sprawled on the sofa, the chairs, and the floor. The living room belongs to Katie's parents and a DANA meeting is in full swing. Our affluent suburban high school frowns on cliques and has organized several dozen intramural clubs, hoping to discourage what the administration considers an erosion of the scholastic social fabric. But in a school as large as ours, segmentation is inevitable, and somewhere in our sophomore year, our class begins to organize itself in extramural clubs. The

Sorelles is the first; a dozen of the school's most popular girls begin wearing lavalieres proclaiming their sisterhood. Soon there is the CABs (letters secret), and the NBAs (secret, of course), and the DANAs. Our letters don't stand for anything which we think is wonderfully witty—an anti-snobbish joke. Necklaces and monogrammed sweatshirts identify the societies, and regardless of the group to which we belong, each of us holds our club sisters almost dearer than family.

Katie's mother has prepared New York cheesecake. I have never tasted anything as heavenly, and years later I still remember how wonderful it is to be in that room, savoring the sour cream topping and sharing the evening with close friends.

I have thought since, that if we could have had a peeping tube into the future on that evening, few of us would have been able to get out of bed the next morning and face our lives.

We would have, between us, twenty-two children, although one of us would know the disappointment of infertility and would have children through adoption. We would have grandchildren numbering in the dozens. Two would become widows while still in their thirties. Five of us would experience divorce. Four of us would remarry. One of us would live with the anguish of a severely handicapped child. One would be diagnosed with multiple sclerosis and would be wheelchair-bound and dependent on round-the-clock nursing help. One of us would develop breast cancer. Two of us would go bald—one from chemotherapy and one from alopecia. For reasons the rest of us never understood, three of us would become estranged from the DANAs and from anything else related to high school.

But on that night in Katie's living room, we are young, we are pretty, and we are enjoying each other. And we can't know what the future holds—neither the terrors nor the incomparable joys that will more than balance them.

As we enter our fifties, we begin gathering every other year. On a specified Friday afternoon, Karen, Lyn, Jan, Joyce, Linda, Sally, and I meet in New York's LaGuardia airport and commandeer two taxis to take us across the river to East End Avenue and Katie's apartment. After the first DANA invasion, Katie's husband prudently takes himself somewhere else for the weekend. Presumably he pokes his nose back into the apartment on Sunday evening and sniffs the complex scent of leftover mingled perfumes from the half dozen women who've been camping there.

Katie is a graceful and generous hostess and her apartment, with its view of the river, is capacious enough to absorb and accommodate the greatest of all slumber parties. Time and place vanish for forty-eight hours and we are the girls again. Our English homework is due on Monday—the usual two dozen vocabulary words—and there's a chemistry test to study for, but for now, it's the weekend and we're free.

This year I make my appearance under Tia, carrying Josie in a plastic bag in my suitcase and with a shiny, bald dome to display to my old schoolmates. If I'd been thirty-years-old instead of sixty-two, I'm not sure I would have made my plane reservation, but now at twice thirty, I am eager for the experience.

"Is it Josie?" Katie cries when I enter her bedroom. I have written her letters sharing the steps of my process and telling her about purchasing the glam wig on the internet. I have written, wittily I hope, about the flurry of compliments Josie has drawn.

"Actually, it's Tia."

It feels very comfortable to go turtle in the company of the DANAs. Bald is who I am right now and with these women especially, there can be no secrets.

BIRTHDAY CANDLES

Two birthday cakes are presented to me this year. The first is baked by my daughter. She brings it proudly to her coffee table, candles flickering, and sets it down with a flourish.

"Ah, ah," Liz interjects as I take a deep breath and prepare to blow. "You have to make a wish, you know."

I pause and wish for hair. Then, with Don, Liz, and Paul watching, I finish drawing the breath and expel it over the cake, moving my entire upper body counterclockwise in order to hit every candle with air. The last two flicker, then begin to glow with new enthusiasm as if fed on the oxygen.

Liz's face is twisted in horror as her eyes meet mine.

"I know what you wished," she breathes.

How funny to feel superstitious. But I *do* feel superstitious and I know Liz certainly does. I laugh; it is a mask for disappointment.

"Now who wants some cake?" I ask gaily.

It's two weeks later and I've been given an opportunity to redeem my wish. My friend Mary has produced a surprise birthday cake. Mary and John have a birthday cake tradition that mandates the celebrant must remain silent until the cake is cut, served all around and the first piece eaten.

Mary places the cake—all swirls of meringue and pink writing—in front of me and John reminds me, unnecessarily, of the silence tradition.

"Now make a wish and blow," they coach.

I pride myself on my lung capacity. I've never smoked a cigarette, have been able to swim fair distances underwater, work out regularly and practice martial arts. It is nothing; I re-tell my wish to myself, draw in my breath and release it.

A single candle stands lighted like a beacon.

I am careful to maintain the silence as I busily cut and serve my birthday cake. What portent have these candles foretold? Do they speak the truth? Will I really remain hairless for the year to come?

LOCKS OF LOVE

My niece Molly has gone to Grenada with the Peace Corps and with her husband David. Letters, photos, but especially emails zing back and forth between the Caribbean and Massachusetts. Molly's older sister Abby is disgusted by the pictures of Molly's long blonde hair. Too long and too hot for the tropics, Abby pronounces, so when Molly and David head home for their mid-assignment break, Abby makes an appointment for Molly's hair to be cut.

"You can get rid of that nuisance mop," Abby proclaims, "and some unfortunate child will benefit through Locks of Love."

Molly's blonde hair reaches halfway down her back, but she takes it to a designated Locks of Love hairdresser in Chicopee and is shorn.

The organization called Locks of Love was founded by Madonna Coffman, a retired cardiac nurse, who developed alopecia in her twenties—the result, apparently—of a hepatitis vaccination. Fifteen years later, she recovered but ironically her four-year-old daughter lost all her hair. Difficult as it had been for Madonna to lose her hair, she says that her daughter's loss was much harder. Her daughter ultimately recovered, but in the meantime, Mrs. Coffman had turned her full-time attention to Locks of Love.

Locks of Love is a non-profit organization that provides wigs and hairpieces to children eighteen years or younger who are experiencing long-term medical hair loss. LOL refers to these hairpieces in the medical terminology as cranial prosthesis.

LOL volunteers screen potential prosthesis candidates, giving primary consideration to those with family financial need and documented medical diagnosis of long-term hair loss. Hair salons generously sprinkled throughout every state and Canada participate in the program, so donors can easily locate a place to "contribute" their hair.

The Locks of Love Web site explains the program in good detail and features photos of recipients and donors, as well as a list of participating hair salons.

Molly's new hair cut just brushes the tips of her ears.

"Do you miss your old hair?" I ask.

Molly gives her head a flick, a gesture that previously would have sent a rope of hair flipping back and forth across each shoulder.

"Yeah, I guess I do, but it's doing more good now than it did for me."

COMPENSATING

"I am a big believer in make-up," Dr. Chapin states. (This is wonderful to hear a dermatologist say.)

"And good earrings," I add.

When your appearance is compromised by baldness, you have to be vigilant about other areas of personal appearance. And so I learn to be careful about applying makeup each morning, and no matter what, to plug in pretty earrings.

ASSUMPTIONS

"It'll grow back. I promise. Mine did."

The woman in the supermarket line, seeing my shiny sidewalls, is grinning confidently at me.

I draw a deep breath, exhale carefully, and place a bagful of spinach and a clutch of grapes on the conveyor belt. How can you be so sure? I want to snap.

She mistakes my sigh for discouragement and continues her cheerleading.

"I'm a survivor, too," she confides. "You'll have hair again in no time, you'll see."

Her assurance annoys me, but I'm getting used to it. People look at me and make assumptions.

"Nice to see you hair grow back! You all better now yes?" The cheerful Korean man in the dry cleaner's shop is complimenting my wig.

I explain.

His cheerful expression turns rueful.

"Oh. So sorry, so sorry."

One day in the mail I receive a handmade bead bracelet from a woman I hardly know but who has obviously gotten a look at me.

"I will pray for you as you go through your treatments," reads the note enclosed with the bracelet.

I struggle to remember that these assumptions are well intended. It wouldn't do, I think, to give a tart answer but sometimes I am tempted to shout. "Don't assume! You don't know anything about this!"

My hair may not grow back and cheerful assurances from strangers that it will is irritating.

When my friend Ann was diagnosed with breast cancer, I was concerned for her. She braved the chemotherapy and donned a cancer wig and I followed her progress with hope and concern. We sat in church services together, two bald women under hair that was not homegrown. Then came the Sunday, less than a year after her diagnosis, that Ann didn't wear a wig. From five pews back I observed that she had her own, real hair. It was short, to be sure, but damn it, it was her own! I was almost as pleased as if it had been mine. But it wasn't mine. And while I cheered Ann's achievement, I couldn't completely control my envy. I'd been bald more than a year before Ann's diagnosis, and I'm *still* bald, while she has a lovely headful of strawberry blonde curls.

Will the day come for me when I can sit in church with my own real hair?

NOSE HAIR

If there is ever an indelicate subject, it is surely nose hair. As I write this, I think of my late mother—a great arbiter of the vulgar versus the tasteful—and she surely would be disappointed in me right now. But it is a fact of life, nose hair, so here we go.

It took a while for me to realize I didn't have any. My first reaction to the discovery was: "Oh boy! One more kind of unwanted hair that I don't have to worry about controlling."

I put nose hair in the same category as armpit hair, you see. Now, however, I've subtracted it out of that classification.

Without nasal hair, I feel open to risk for more-than-my share of viral infections, so I am taking a few precautions; I'm using a saline spray, taking a daily multivitamin, and touching wood.

Nose hair is a perfect little filtration system for straining out airborne germs, dust, and foreign materials.

It also traps material trying to go the other way. Without nose hair, my nose runs constantly. When I walk the dog on cold mornings I am forced to keep a wad of tissue pressed to my face, and yesterday—completely fed up with the drippage—I stuffed wads of cotton up both nostrils. That worked just fine—until we encountered another dog walker. Do I explain this? I wondered as we drew closer to each other, or do I follow Queen Victoria's approach of never apologize, never explain. Within ten feet of the fellow walker, I opted for the royal treatment, delivered a small, regal wave and swept grandly past.

EMOTIONAL ISSUES

Hair is a highly charged emotional issue. Think of the last time you were at the hairdresser's getting a disastrous haircut or a coloring treatment that was clearly going sour. You know that in the fullness of time, the cut or the color is going to grow out, but just for a moment, recall how you felt sitting in that chair regarding the mayhem that is happening on your head—a botch-job that you will have to live with intimately for several weeks at least. Moreover, you may be headed for an important social engagement *this very night* that will be ruined by this tonsorial mistake; the promise of eventual correction is little consolation.

Now try to consider how you'd feel if all your hair came out. All of it. Suddenly. And not only that, what if there were no promise of regrowth?

This is what confronts a woman facing chemotherapy for breast cancer. This is what confronts people who have received a diagnosis of alopecia areata totalis universalis. It's no wonder that instances of low self esteem, depression, and anxiety are common among both groups.

For many women who receive the breast cancer diagnosis, hair loss is the immediate and most compelling issue.

"Will I lose my hair?"

"Will I *have to* lose my hair?"

As they brush against the possibility of losing life, many women focus on hair loss. It is a big—a very big—issue. Perhaps hair is a metaphor for life itself. And its loss is the tangible proof of a silent and insidious disease that is otherwise invisible and undetectable.

I've known women whose first act, upon receiving the breast cancer diagnosis, has been to have their hair cut and constructed into a wig so they could comfortably continue to wear their very own hair during the bald spell that would accompany their months of cancer treatment. "Hair therapy" is one of the treatments a sensitive oncologist uses to treat patients.

A cancer patient, at least, can understand what is about to happen to her. A person with an alopecia diagnosis may not have that luxury, if you can call it that. For an alopecia sufferer, the road is much darker, much less clear. How much hair will be lost? Will it ever grow back?

Several years ago, a few shocking (to me) statistics on alopecia sufferers were published in the British paper *The Guardian*. The paper claimed that forty-eight percent of Alopecians admitted they had considered suicide. Sixty-eight percent stated that their jobs had been destroyed. And forty percent claimed their marriages had been disrupted.

When the National Alopecia Foundation states that alopecia is life changing, they are right on the money.

So what is an Alopecian to do?

The answer for me is: the best you can.

At some point I had to decide that I am not my hair. This seems obvious when you say it, but the deep-dish belief in the truth of the statement may be harder to get a purchase on.

A man I knew some years ago was laid off from his job. He had a young wife, a baby, and a brand new mortgage, and the sudden severance from his company emotionally crippled him for a time. He had worked in a large firm and had a position that only had meaning in the context of that company. His title was basically techno-babble. He'd never had a hard-and-fast job description like "carpenter" or "physical therapist"—some title that described a trade or bestowed professional credibility. For his whole, short life as a salary-earner, he had thought of himself—had defined himself—in the context of his company. His abrupt separation was tantamount to an amputation.

Well, Larry recovered, of course, picked himself up, and went on to a new and more lucrative situation, but there were many dark days when he literally sat in a chair and didn't know who he was. At that point in his life, he had not separated his ego from his occupation.

Likewise, most folks have never had to separate their self-images from the hair on their own heads.

Much of my experience with alopecia areata has centered on coping mechanisms—the handling of the emotional issues that accompany dramatic hair loss. Writing has been therapeutic. This is understandable since I've made my living writing. A pen in my hand or a keyboard under my fingers has been a direct link with the part of my mind that deals with emotion and will. My writing implements have been tools of emotional exploration and the simple task of forming letters, words, and sentences has given me perspective and a needed emotional outlet.

I have made the decision to cope with this disease as gracefully and bravely as I can. This attitude is not guaranteed to come with a diagnosis, however. For me it was a conscious and sometimes difficult choice. I could add myself into *The Guardian*'s statistics by considering suicide or I could allow alopecia to shake my marriage to its very roots. That my marriage is still sound is due in no small measure to Don's steadfastness, as well as my own hard work.

"I'll bet you never thought you'd have a bald wife," I say, as I lay my head on the pillow next to his.

"I miss your pretty hair," he admits loyally, "but you still look beautiful to me."

I don't have to believe him, of course. It is my choice to believe him. I could choose another approach and could say: "That is just Irish blarney." Or I could think: "Oh sure, that's what he says, but I know what he is thinking, and he is thinking, 'She is sooo ugly!'" But I am happy to say I make the responsible choice here, too, and I am able to smile confidently at him and simply say, "Thank you."

It is a big responsibility, being an Alopecian. It is an on-going mental game of choice. A constant test of mental mettle.

FAILING

Kell regards my head with perplexity. It's been two weeks since my last appointment, and he is getting his first chance to see that I've lost a considerable amount of hair.

"What is going on?" he wants to know.

Why do they all ask this, these health care professionals? How am I supposed to know?

I immediately revert into the eager-to-please student of years ago and attempt to explain the unexplainable by sort of apologizing for the hair loss.

Now, lying on the table with needles sprouting out of various parts of me, I scold myself for this need-to-please attitude and for my feelings of failure. I've lost more hair, therefore I've failed. I'm supposed to be *growing hair*, not losing it. I'm letting down my team (that is, the dermatologist and the acupuncturist) as they work their therapies on me. I am not playing by the rules of this get-better game.

With my eyes closed and George Winston's "Winter into Spring" music dripping into my ears, I review this realization.

I suppose I could take the opposite approach and blame the treatment and the therapist. Maybe it is the acupuncture treatment and the topical irritation therapy that is failing *me*. But I was raised to be a polite girl; I would hate to have Kell or Dr. Chapin think I believed that. Better to take the responsibility for failure upon myself.

SUMMER

BALD AS A BEAN

BURNING THE BEAN

Five hours in the rain driving home from Maine and I'm tired. How good the lights of the house look through the cheerless drizzle. The carriage lamps are all wearing halos of mist. Don has been careful to turn on every welcoming light he can find and has even lighted some candles in the fireplace. I've only been gone two nights to visit Jan in Stonington, but I know I was missed. Don has dinner ready—his own spaghetti sauce, which requires three hours of preparation including a slow, artistic chopping of each and every vegetable.

Exhausted, I anticipate the luxury of my own bed, and because I've been away from my routine of irritation therapy, I decide to be dutiful in its application.

In the night something doesn't feel right, but I'm groggy and I can't be bothered figuring out what is troubling me. Too hot. I pull off my white cotton nightcap and toss it on the quilt.

One look in the mirror in the morning and I know the worst. My head has turned the red-brown burned-blueberry-barren look I recognize. Furthermore, I am feeling feverish. And wouldn't this just be Sunday! I doubt dermatologists have emergency services.

So when Dr. Chapin's office opens Monday morning, mine is the first call. I ask to speak to Judy, Dr. Chapin's nurse and give her an embarrassed account of my mistake.

"I put the wrong medication on my head," I tell her. "I used the one that I'm only supposed to leave on for fifteen minutes. Except I left it on all night."

Judy promises to get back to me as fast as she can, and she is good as her word. Dr. Chapin phones in a prescription ointment and leaves orders to lay-off the topicals.

My poor head looks like it was roasted on the end of a stick in a campfire. I am such a mess that I can't face Kell for an acupuncture treatment. I call and explain my dilemma.

"It really doesn't bother me, you know," he says mildly.

"But it bothers *me*. I just feel too ghastly to face anyone. I'll call and set up another appointment when this burn is gone and the scabs go away."

PRIMARY CARE

In order to keep my appointments with Dr. Chapin, I have to get regular dispensations from my primary care physician. These are the rules of the HMO. Dr. Tyler's office is generous about these referrals, but for most of my treatments for alopecia areata, Dr. Tyler is in the dark.

"How many treatments will you need?" asks the referral writer in Dr. Tyler's office after I explain I am being treated by Dr. Chapin for alopecia areata.

"Ah, I have no idea," I say. And I haven't.

She is kind. "I will write you up for four," she says. "And by the way, you haven't seen Dr. Tyler for quite a while."

Well, she is right about that, so to keep things squared up nicely, I make an appointment with my primary care physician.

Suddenly the game rules shift.

"Is this an emergency?" the appointment maker wants to know.

"Honestly, no."

"Oh." I hear the sound of pages flipping and the voice on the phone announces an appointment that is a full five months away. This takes me aback. Something devilish in me wants to shock her. "I don't a have a single hair on my body. While this may not be an emergency to you, it gets *my* attention."

But I simply write down the appointment date and time and say thank you.

So today, as I am shown into Dr. Tyler's examining room, I reflect that it has been five months since I made my appointment for a routine check-up. And Dr. Tyler reminds me when he swings in, that it has been a long time since we've had a professional meeting. But that's okay. I see my GYN regularly, am dutiful about mammograms and bone density scans.

"You look good," he says cheerfully.

"You think so?"

For dramatic effect, I sweep Tia off my head, revealing my highly polished dome. Dr. Tyler seems keenly interested and not at all alarmed or put off. Dr. Chapin is a colleague and he wants to know the details of my treatment. I mention my idea that this trouble was triggered by Lyme disease.

"I look at it this way," I say. "Lyme is known to cause rheumatoid arthritis in some cases, right? Rheumatoid arthritis is an autoimmune disease. If Lyme can be responsible for one sort of autoimmune disease, why wouldn't it trigger others as well?"

Dr. Tyler rubs his chin in an intrigued sort of way. "Could be possible," he admits. His curiosity is stirred.

"While you slip into a johnny, let me do a quick bit of sleuthing."

He comes back to thump my knee and listen to me breathe. "Couldn't find anything on that one quick pass, but I'll keep looking."

After my blood has been drawn for standard tests and I am on the way out of the office, Dr. Tyler is still sleuthing. "Nothing seems to be written up," he says.

"You can be the first," I tell him generously. "Publish it in *The New England Journal of Medicine* and be famous."

Dr. Tyler looks me squarely in the eye. "It's a funny disease, alopecia," he says. "I've seen people go along for two years or five years without growing a single hair, and then bingo! It comes back fast. Like someone has turned on a light."

Comforting words to me. I leave his office feeling happy and encouraged.

EYEBROW TATTOOS

This is ridiculous! Each morning I painstakingly draw eyebrows on my face, only to have them erased by my own skin oils within an hour. Grumbling, I go searching on the web for a better way. Maybe I'll look again at false eyebrows.

My quest turns up tattoos. I had always thought eyebrow tattoos were permanent marks rendered in ink by a sometime artist in a sleazy tattoo parlor, but they turn out to be temporary transfers that last from three to five days. For a mere four dollars, I can own a half-dozen sets of these. And among the places to buy them is my favorite online supplier, Headcovers.com.

Nothing is easy.

First, I have to decide what style and color to buy. There are various lengths, degrees of thickness, arched brows and straight ones. But for four dollars, I figure I can't go far wrong.

Don helps me apply the first set.

"How do we do this? What do the directions say?"

"We're supposed to peel off this backing material."
Don is reading from the little instruction booklet. "Then
we place the brows against your face ... is this where you
want them?"

"How can I tell? I can't really see because your hand
is in the way ... yes, yes, that's fine."

"Well, hold them in place while I get a facecloth
wet. Now you hold the facecloth on the brows for a few
seconds. Okay. Take the cloth away and here, we peel off
the papers and ... hey! They look great."

And they did. A little redder in color than any hair
I've ever grown, but not bad ... not bad at all.

Confident in our success, I attempt the second
application solo. The right brow looks fine but I've gotten
the left one too close to the bridge of my nose and the effect
is bizarre. I erase the offending brow with Vaseline and try
again. The result is the same, but what the hell, for two
days, I wear my lopsided tattoos which give me a vaguely
cross-eyed air, but most of my vanity has vanished with
my hair, so I don't care.

READY WHEN YOU ARE
Do not push the river; it will flow by itself. Lao-tse

Suddenly all the treatments I have been taking for this alopecia areata thing seem ludicrous. Dr. Chapin and Kell and yes, even I, have been focusing on my head. Herbs and needles, injections and unguents, massage and multivitamins, and the detested Rogaine for Women ... are all designed to wake up the hair follicles and cause hair to grow *on my head!*

Hey, guys ... what about the rest of me? I don't have hair anywhere on my body!

No one seems to care about those other, less-public body parts. Well, why not, I want to know?

In one of those moments of epiphany, I've decided the treatments on my scalp seem silly. Time and money and hocus-pocus—we've done everything but burn fingernail pairings under the light of the new moon.

And so I've got a new theory now. And it's been under my nose all along. In fact, I've been preaching it.

When my body is ready to grow hair and support it—in other words, when my body is finished with alopecia areata—then new hair will grow. It will grow all over my body—on my head, on my legs and inside my nose. It will grow under my arms and I will have to take up shaving again, drat it. It will grow on my brow bones and I will throw away my eyebrow tattoos. I will have to get it cut (or shaved). I'll have to buy shampoo for it and new brushes and combs. I will buy crème rinse again and a new hair dryer and will start spending money every month to keep my hair groomed. I'll take it out to beauty salons for stylings, and I'll let the wind blow through it in convertibles and boats. Sheaves of it will fall across my cheek again when I bend to lift the garage door, and when I lie down at night, a thick wave of it will once more fan across the pillow and Don, looking over from his neighboring pillow, will see only a tousle of silky hair and maybe the curve of a real eyebrow.

Now it is entirely possible that my body will never decide to kick alopecia areata. In which case, I will remain hairless for the rest of my days. I picture myself as an old lady in a rest home and decide I'd just as soon be bald as be subjected to the weekly ministrations of a hairdresser who styles the same cap of lavender-rinsed fragile curls on all the female residents of the home.

PARTING

I am ushered into Dr. Chapin's examining room with remarkable promptness. And even more remarkably, the doctor herself makes her entrance while I am still reading an article on the ten common food myths.

"Well, well, well, what have we here?"

"Nothing much," I reply. "Just a few light patches of hair where the cortisone was injected."

I turn so she can inspect the back of my head.

"No, not much," she agrees.

We sit and face each other. Dr. Chapin takes the little wheeled stool that can scoot all over the office, and I seat myself on the examining room's single chair instead of on my usual perch on the end of the exam table. We have both reached the same conclusions and now the only thing to do is figure out how to share those conclusions without injuring the other party; thus will we validate each other.

The treatments have obviously failed. Or more precisely, I have failed to respond to the treatments. We both know it is impractical to try more cortisone injections. If that protocol were going to work, the eight injections would have generated hair all over my head by now. I envision a grid of one-square-inch cells drawn on my skull with eyebrow pencil and having Dr. Chapin jam a needle into the center of each cell. Too much cortisone. Too much trouble. Too many skull dents or dells. Neither of us would even consider it.

I offer my "when my body is ready" theory and she doesn't dispute it. We agree, then, to allow my body the space and time to decide if it wants to reject the alopecia areata. If it does, then I will visit her again in six months. In the meantime she reminds me I can continue the topical treatments at my discretion. Or not. I choose the "or not." Like the cortisone shots, the topicals appear to have done nothing.

Dr. Chapin regards me with a clear gaze. "You have a nice face," she states. "Your skin is good; you have lovely cheekbones and beautiful lips. And you seem to be managing well with your hairpiece. So ..." and she stands and puts out her hand in an offer to shake mine. "I'll see you in January. In the meantime, call if you need anything—prescription refills or anything. And the best of luck."

January. On this July day, the pit of winter seems forever-off.

I recall the day ten months ago in Dr. Chapin's office when I had applied for help because I was losing my hair. If I had known then that I would be bald as a bean by the following July and would be dismissed into the world with nothing more that could be done, I would have been devastated beyond description. But I had not known, and so, along the way had adjusted to a condition that I could hardly have contemplated. Bald as a bean, I found I could be calm and comfortable. Dr. Chapin and I had given it our best. The rest was going to be up to me—or more accurately, up to my body. The decision to reverse the autoimmune process rests now solely with the old bod. And that's okay.

I leave Dr. Chapin's office with a light step and trot down the four flights to the parking lot. The dark glass doors that I pass reveal a trim woman in linen trousers and a tailored white shirt, short, gold-tipped hair, small pearl earrings. The picture of health to anyone who doesn't know I have no hair.

A LETTER

To Martin Kelly, I write a letter:

I have been thinking about you recently. It has occurred to me that I have sunk below your radar and I feel you deserve an explanation. (It has also occurred to me that I may flatter myself too much to think you have noticed my disappearance, or that you might care, and if that's the case, just disregard this letter, which I suspect is going to get out of hand anyway.)

You may recall that our last communication centered on an appointment that I cancelled because I'd applied the wrong medication to my scalp. I said that I'd get back to you when the burns subsided. Well, the burns have subsided and I want to tell you what has happened; then I'm going to tell you what I have decided to do.

Dr. Chapin has given me six more cortisone shots, which she hoped would excite the follicles on my head so that my whole scalp would bloom with hair. What happened instead was six small, anemic-looking patches of down. This past week, when I presented these to her inspection, she and I sat down and I had the satisfaction of hearing her speak the conclusions I had been slowing drawing for a month.

I've grown to believe that the attempts to grow hair on my head make no sense at all. I have alopecia areata totalis universalis (total hair loss over the entire body). Why all this concern about the head? I realized that when my body is ready to give up alopecia areata, then hair will grow on my head, on my eyebrows, in my nose, on my legs and with my luck on my chin! I have decided I am quite content to wait for this to happen. And if it never does, then I'm okay with that, too.

So Dr. Chapin and I looked each other in the eye and she said essentially the same thing. I know, from my own research, that she tried every protocol available except prednisone (which I refused to take and which she didn't push). I can continue the topicals if I wish—the stuff I call irritation therapy—or I can leave them alone. I think I'll leave them alone. In six months she and I will see if anything has changed.

I feel oddly free, like a child who's been let out of school early. It's up to me now.

Now in the scheme of treatment, I believe acupuncture has a place. While it is true that my chi wasn't stimulated enough to wake up the sleeping hair follicles, it still seems that acupuncture is of value. For budgetary reasons, however, I am going to continue my break from treatment. I had allowed myself a certain number of sessions and I exceeded that number slightly. I hope, however, to return to treatment when I think my body may be getting ready to stop enjoying its fling with alopecia areata.

Yours in gratitude for all you've done for me.

THE EXPERT

Martha catches up with me after church.

"Could I have a word with you about a medical matter?"

Mystified, I follow her into the relative quiet of the church parlor, where she turns to face me.

"Emily's losing her hair. It's coming out in clumps."

Emily is one of Martha's daughters—the other is Abigail—but I can't tell the girls apart. Both are tall and lean with manes of hair and straight, bright teeth. Even when they are dressed up, they look like they are posing with tennis rackets just after a game.

"Is it falling out at the roots or just breaking off?

"Oh, it's not breaking," Martha is firm. "It's coming out at the roots. Why? What does that mean?"

"I haven't the faintest idea, really." I smile. "I just remember that's the first question Dr. Chapin asked me."

"Interesting." Martha draws the word out, giving it several extra syllables, and she scribbles this question in a little spiral notebook cupped in her palm.

"The doctor has been doing tests and one showed a higher than normal amount of testosterone in her blood, but the next time they tested, it came back normal."

"Thyroid?" I asked. "Have they tested for that?"

"Oh yes," Martha says quickly, "and that appears normal, too, although Emily does have some other symptoms of hyperthyroid."

"Well, I have alopecia areata," I explain. "All my tests for endocrinology stuff came back perfectly normal, but alopecia is an autoimmune disease and ..."

"Wait," Martha begs, "spell that."

I obligingly spell alopecia areata and she carefully copies this down.

"I think it's best to learn as much as you can, don't you?" Her eyes hold mine earnestly.

I remember my reluctance to Google and while I agree you should learn as much as you can, I don't think you should try to learn it faster than you can emotionally assimilate it. No point in scaring yourself to death. I hope Martha doesn't start telling Emily about me. To tell a twenty-three-year-old woman that she is about to become as bald as a bean would be like handing her a load of bricks—a load far heavier than she could bear, and one that she might never need to hold.

I scratch furiously in my mind for some scrap of sound, helpful information I can give Martha that is, at the same time, positive.

"A lot of people have symptoms of alopecia areata," is what I come up with. "For most, it is a temporary condition and the hair grows back. Many people just lose a small amount of hair. Cases as extreme as mine are rare.

I suggest that Martha and Emily might want to consult Dr. Chapin, saying that she is an excellent physician for this sort of problem, but I have to give an ironic laugh as I do so. "Not that she could do anything for *me*, but she says she sees cases like mine about once a year, if that. She apparently sees several cases a month of people with mild cases of hair loss"

I assure Martha that Dr. Chapin is well respected and I think Emily would benefit from seeing a specialist in hair problems—that is, a dermatologist.

I wish Martha and Emily sincere good luck, but the conversation haunts me all day as I imagine a beautiful young woman terrified at the prospect of dramatic, or even insignificant, hair loss. My mind races over the "whys" and "what-ifs" and "what-thens" that Emily and Martha are surely tilting at. How much information should I give? Too much may be more harmful than not enough. I'm beginning to appreciate Dr. Chapin's position, remembering how she trod very cautiously that fine path between knowledge and terror. I'm beginning to see that the emotional terrain differs from patient to patient, and the diagnosing physician has to make a guess-timate about just how much each patient can be safely told.

But it troubles me to be the resource for someone who is losing hair. I am an example of maximal hair loss. I am a picture of just how bad it can be, and in most cases, the loss won't be nearly so extreme. I don't want my example to frighten people, but somehow I want to let them know that even in the most extreme cases, the news isn't all that bad—or it doesn't have to be if you can find ways of coping or if you are fortunate enough to find a treatment that works.

A HAIR!

A hair! An actual hair! And it's on my earlobe! An offspring, clearly, of the old rogue follicle that used to regularly send out an aberrant hair about the gauge of a 0.002 wire. Fastening a pearl earring to my lobe I come upon this hair and greet it joyously like an old friend. In the past, when this horrible single hair manifested, I would tweeze it out instantly. I wonder though, is it a recent growth or simply a coarse survivor of the blight that put all my other follicles to sleep? I am torn between the pleasure of tugging it out and the satisfaction of letting it stand as a possible testament to my sole, productive hair follicle.

In the end, though, I hunt up the long-retired tweezers and slowly extricate the offending hair. Actually, the hair doesn't offend me much. It is offensive only in the sense that well-groomed women do not have hairy earlobes. Still, bowing to social custom, I haul the thing out with a heavy sense of Abraham holding the knife over Isaac. Am I killing the last remaining hair I will ever spawn?

Such melodrama!
There! Out it comes!

BALD AS A BEAN

AUTUMN AGAIN

BALD AS A BEAN

SHOPPING AT COSTCO

"You're going through chemotherapy, aren't you?" the woman says.

I pause, midway through the stack of sweatpants, and with a flash of irritation, interrupt my search for a size six. Irritability erases my charity.

"No."

"Well, I wondered," she says, "because, you know" and here she lowers her voice conspiratorially, "because you don't have any hair ... back there." She makes a waving motion indicating the nape of my neck.

I sigh. I wish I didn't have to explain the situation to some other shopper in Costco—some woman I don't know and will never see again, and now I've lost my place in the stack of sweatpants and will have to begin all over from the top.

"I have alopecia areata."

And then, in response to her blank stare, I have to elaborate. "It's an autoimmune disease that caused me to lose all my hair."

"Oh. Well I'm going through chemotherapy," she offers.

She appears to have a full head of dark wavy hair, and I offer a compliment.

"It's a wig," she explains. "Don't you have a wig?"

"Yes, I have several." My God, my own patience astounds me! "I'd just rather wear a baseball cap much of the time."

"That is so brave of you," she breathes looking awed. Then she turns as her companion urges her, "Gina, look at this darling sweater! Isn't it darling?"

Brave? What a curious adjective. There's nothing brave about it. Simple necessity is all there is to it.

WHAT I LEARNED FROM PETER JENNINGS

When newsman Peter Jennings was diagnosed with lung cancer, he made the courageous decision to announce the diagnosis on national television. He sat in his usual anchor chair, looked straight at the camera and laid his cards on the table. Named his illness in bold tones and said what he was going to do about it—chemotherapy, radiation, and continued work, if possible, even if he felt lousy. Then toward the end of his announcement he said one thing that got to me. He repeated something he'd said to his physician.

"Well, Doc," he said, "when does the hair go?"

I sat there in stunned (and bald) silence. The survival odds of a person with lung cancer aren't good at all. Breast, prostate—some cancers you stand a pretty good chance of beating—but lung cancer isn't one of them. So while Peter Jennings is looking down the barrel, he's concerned about his hair? He's Peter Jennings! He's a guy! His hair?

This gave me some more insight into the trauma of sudden hair loss. It is a big deal emotionally. And not just for women. Not just for me.

THE GIRLS

They wait on their wig stands like a line of wallflowers at a dance: Josie, Tia, Raquel, Chloe, and Jill. When there is a special occasion—a business meeting, a church service, a party, or a restaurant date—one of the girls is chosen. Putting on a wig is like putting on a whole new personality.

Josie: She is an ash blonde with highlighted tips. Short, chic, and tailored, she is usually picked to attend church service and business meetings. Josie is the good girl, the proper lady.

Tia: Also a frost-tipped ash blonde, Tia is cropped even shorter than Josie. Tia wears jeans and loves casual events. She can be combed out with ruffling fingers and never minds if a gust of wind attacks; she emerges unscathed.

Raquel: The biker chick. Her honey-blonde hair stands up all over the top in spikes. Raquel is perfect with a pair of jeans—tight jeans—and a leather jacket. My son was intrigued when he met Raquel; kept thinking he knew

her from somewhere but couldn't quite place her. Finally
he had it. "I know who you look like," he cried. "You look
like Kevin Bacon in Footloose!" My friend John was less
charitable. "What," he exclaimed when he met her, "do you
have on your head?" But never mind. Raquel is Don's
favorite date and Don is the person who matters most.

Chloe: Well, doesn't everyone want to be a platinum
blonde at least for one day? Chloe is my chance. Chloe is
ultimate glam. She is frivolous. She is high maintenance.
And she doesn't get invited out much, mainly because her
alter ego (me) doesn't get many invitations to glamorous
places.

Jill: Jill is the younger sister of Josie. Don can't tell
these girls apart. And Jill is a testament to my tendency to
settle into familiar ruts on the road. After decades of
pageboy-wearing, I have apparently shifted to a short swing-
back style and can't be shoved out of it.

Don has entered into the spirit of wig-wearing with
good sportsmanship. Sometimes, with an event shaping
up, I'll invite him to choose the woman he wants to take
out for the evening. He is especially fond of Raquel but I
think she is unsuitable for a number of venues. Too raffish.

In my career as an Alopecian, I have come across
many names to substitute for the word wig. Apparently
there is something crass about the word, maybe because it
brings to mind a justice of the British system or a powdered
seventeenth century dandy. Unit was Humberto's word of
choice. Hairpiece is a common term. The Locks of Love
people say cranial prosthesis. And rug is a rude old slang
expression everybody has heard. I don't mind the word wig
but I prefer to think of the row of personalities in my closet
simply as The Girls.

HOPE WITHOUT EXPECTATION

Autumn again and there isn't much to write about that hasn't already been said. The business of sudden hair loss is past and my baldness is just a normal day-to-day fact. So this chapter in my saga is short.

I've stopped dreaming about growing hair. I can't tell just when the dreams stopped, I only know it has been quite a while since I've dreamed of standing in the shower and reaching for a razor to shave my legs. I can't remember the last time I dreamed about brushing my hair, leaning over from the waist the way I used to do to give the underside of my mane its hundred strokes. I used to be so savage in my brushing; so ruthless. And so casual about its thickness.

I still remember what it felt like to have a swoop of hair brush my cheek and cover my right eye every time I bent to lift the garage door. I still recall settling into my pillow each night and allowing the matching swoop on the left side to fall over my left eye and across my cheek. The memories are still intact but the reality is gaining influence and power over the memory. The way my hair moved and was lives only as a ghost thing. I miss it but I do not mourn.

It's been nearly one year now since I parted with Dr. Chapin and wrote a farewell letter to Martin Kelly. My topical ointments are packed away in a bottom drawer. There may be a time I will dig them out and return to the complex regime of treating my scalp. But I doubt it. I have settled a few emotional issues about myself and alopecia areata and this is the big one: I would like to have hair. I can accept that I don't. I can hope to grow hair—to recover from this autoimmune disease, or at least to send it into remission—but I have stopped counting the days and weeks until that happens. I have come to accept that it may never happen. I may end my days as I began them—bald as a bean. So I have hope but not much expectation.

So ... a few more hats, a few more wigs, a few more jokes ...

AFTERWARD

It's been nearly a year since I recorded the last casual essay in the chapter called *Autumn Again*. With yet another autumn just a calendar page away, I find I'm finally getting hair back. And it isn't through the miracle of modern medicine or the magic of alternative therapies. It is simply because the rapscallion autoimmune disease called alopecia areata is apparently deciding to release its hold on my body—*for the time being.*

My eyelashes grew back so gradually I didn't notice their coming. It was my friend Mary, sitting next to me in a theater, who remarked with surprise, "Hey! You've got lashes!"

And so I did.

Were there as many as I'd had before? Were they as thick? How odd that I couldn't answer those questions. I just didn't know.

Some women would have dashed out and bought a tube of mascara to celebrate their new eyelashes, but I ignored mine. If I made too much of them, would they disappear just to spite my enthusiasm?

Next my eyebrows began to grow—fine hairs of no discernable color began to sprout—and I could see that the eyebrows were much lower than the ones I had been designing with my pencil and pasting on with tattoos. Taking a clue from these new hairs, I filled in brows with a khaki color and realized I had gained a much more realistic look than the weird, surprised expression I'd been wearing for a year and a half.

Now a fine down of hair has sprouted on the left side of my head. If I turn my head just right so the light catches the hairs, I can see them. But what color are they? No color. The color of vodka. There are champagne blondes, why not vodka-locks?

But I have to grin at the antics of the old trickster alopecia. When hair comes back it only grows on one side. So the joke continues.

At my request, Don takes the eyebrow pencil and traces around the hair patches. I want to see the patterns. I want to establish some kind of high water marks for the new growth. I still appear quite bald, but no matter. I know the hair is there. It is growing and it will reveal itself in the fullness of its own time.

So perhaps the disease is reversing. And perhaps it isn't. It is a tease, this disease of alopecia areata is. I will just have to wait and see.

The irony of writing about new growth as autumn nears isn't lost on me. I still have hold-over feelings about my Seasons Theory.

And there is another irony.

As I write this, the Norway maple in the backyard will soon be deciduating yellow leaves into the grass and gutters in the annual autumnal ritual, but the sugar maple on the front lawn has succumbed to black rot—a common disease of sugar maples apparently. Many of its limbs are bare; the leaves it sheds aren't the juicy yellow ones of years past but brown ones, dried and curled like old gloves that have worn and stiffened and finally lost their grip. The tree trunk is thick with lichen the color of a coating on a sick tongue.

So things change. I know that better with each passing day, each turning season. Things grow and die. They come and go. They ebb and flow. We will let the sugar maple stand through the winter (if storms don't take it down) and in spring, when the other trees are puffing out with new leaves, we'll call the tree company to take it down. This fall I mark the third anniversary of my private deciduation. I am recovering apparently but the sugar maple is not.

If I ever have a crop of hair again, I plan to keep my new hair brutally short and I intend to find a barber who will run a clipper over my pate every two weeks or so. I have two reasons for this decision. First, I have grown used to the ease of baldness during my years with alopecia areata. After years of hair abuse—of coloring and curling and of washing and blowing, of trimming and fuming and looking longingly at hair styles not my own—it is a relief to rub my wet, bald head with a towel and go on my way. When I wanted to look well turned out, I turned to one of the "girls"—to Raquel or Josie—to confer instant personality and style. I learned to like the convenience and the character shifts.

But there is a second reason for keeping this new hair shorn. Alopecia areata is a capricious disease, capable of flaring up as suddenly as it did the first time. Maybe I don't want to become too attached to my new hair—too invested in it. Maybe the gods will hear me celebrating and come swinging back like so many Delilahs to deal me the blow of baldness once again. It could happen. And if it does, I will better know how to deal with it. I may grieve once again but this time I will know what to do.

ACKNOWLEDGEMENTS

This story about my experience of sudden hair loss has turned out to be a pretty slender volume—the sort of publication that vanishes into bookcases, eclipsed by the spines of fatter, bolder books and sometimes you wonder fleetingly whatever happened to that funny little book about baldness. But there it is. And I make no apologies for the book's weight and girth. I've told the story as it happened and for good measure have thrown in an Afterward. But the hair I described in Afterward has vanished, too. An Alopecian's story is never finished I've found out. Hair today and gone tomorrow pretty much sums it up.

Oh well.

For reasons of professional anonymity, I've changed the names of the medical professionals who are featured in this story. I've kept the names of most of the characters, however—some of them may be surprised to recognize themselves here. A few of the folks who appear are braced for their five minutes of semi-fame. Although many people helped me along the way by supplying moral support and kindness, there were some brave souls who were willing to roll up their sleeves, read the manuscript, and give me some feedback. And so I want to thank my old friend and business partner Dick Amsterdam who has been reading what I write (and picking it apart) for thirty years. Jean Amsterdam cast her English teacher's eye over the document and that gave me some comfort. My DANA sisters raised their hands when I asked if anyone would be willing to be a reader; so thanks to Karen Abraham, Lyn Brown, Sally Carlsen, Jan Goudie, Linda Kast, Katie Mandel, and Joyce Simmelink who read drafts and wrote thoughtful comments. Denise Gressley, who has first-hand knowledge of alopecia areata, read *Bean,* and I especially appreciate her remarks and shared experiences. And finally I close this book the way I started it, with special thanks to my caring husband, Don Doyle.

FOUNDATIONS FOR THE FOLLICLE-LY CHALLENGED

If it is any comfort—and to me it isn't much—there are foundations and not-for-profit outfits dedicated to the causes and challenges of hair loss, including the dissemination of information. The following organizations can be reached online:

> NIAMS: National Institute of Arthritis and Musculoskeletal and Skin Diseases, affiliated is the National Institutes of Health, Department of Health & Human Services. www.NIAMS.nih.gov.

> National Center for Complementary and Alternative Medicine Clearinghouse. http:// nccam.nih.gov

> The American Academy of Dermatology. www.aad.org.

National Alopecia Areata Foundation. www.naaf.org.

American Hair Loss Council. www.ahlc.org.

Heralopecia: Women's Hair Loss Information Support Site (an interactive support group and forum just for women). www.heralopecia.com.

For children with long-term medical hair loss, contact Locks of Love. www.locksoflove.org.

In addition, there are online directories, such as www.HairLossDirect.com that list hair loss websites. From these resources it is possible to get information on all types of hair loss, news of treatments and medications, and links to sites that sell hair loss products. My favorites are www.Headcovers.com and www.PaulaYoung.com.

Nancy Parsons is a retired advertising executive. She lives and writes in North Reading, Massachusetts, where she shares an office with her husband Don Doyle (an artist) and with Gwen (a retired racing greyhound).